HEALING LETTERS

A 140 Day Journey of Healthy Living

Angelena Cortello

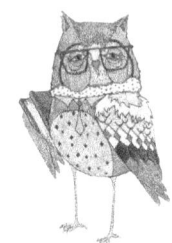

PUBLISHED BY
OUR WRITTEN LIVES OF HOPE, LLC

Our Written Lives of Hope provides publishing services for authors in various educational, religious, and human services organizations. For information, visit ourwrittenlives.com

Copyright © 2015 Angelena Cortello

Library of Congress Cataloging-in-Publication Data
Cortello, Angelena 1979
Healing Letters: A 140 Day Journey of Healthy Living
Library of Congress Control Number: 2015908621
ISBN: 978-1-942923-02-2

Scripture quotations are taken from the King James Version of the Holy Bible, which is in the public domain.

HEALING LETTERS

A 140 Day Journey of Healthy Living

Angelena Cortello

Letter to the Readers

My name is Angelena Cortello, but everyone calls me "Angel."

I had a dream where I was carrying my heavy heart in my hands and the weight of it was hindering my daily life. The people closest to me were standing in a semi-circle in front of me. I asked if they could hold my heart for awhile to give me a break from carrying it since it was so heavy. They agreed to and I gave it to them. They did their best to hold it with the helping healing hands God gave them, but they could only do so much. Eventually, they shook their heads back and forth and handed my heart back to me saying, "We are sorry, but it is too heavy and we do not know what to do with it."

I prayed for the meaning of my dream. I felt the Lord speak to my heart, "They can only hold your heavy heart for so long, until they are unsure what to do with it. They were not meant to know everything about how to handle your heart; only I know what to do with your heart because I am the one who created it."

During my journey I have faced health challenges of addiction, emotional issues and HIV. I desired healing of the areas of my heart that hinder me from living an abundant life. I continuously gave my heart to God one piece at a time, until I could finally trust Him with all of my heart. Now I am gaining healing in many areas of my life from "The Healer."

In this book, I share the healing prayers I have learned through much trial and error. Because I am human, I have to remind myself all of the time to refocus when I get off kilter in some of the areas I discuss. I believe as long as we are connected to God, our Ultimate Healer, practice being as healthy as we can be, and have healthy relationships—then we can live in a victorious manner through any health condition or issue we are challenged with.

Hence, in this 140 Day Journey of Healing Letters to God, I share my heart for Him and the healing ways He has placed in my heart. I hope these prayers, shared in the form of letters to God, will help lead you to inner healing.

This book exposes our thinking and the behavior that hinders us from living the healthy, abundant life God has for each of us. A lot of what I have written about has come from my own personal challenges. I have failed miserably in some of the issues presented. My failures caused me to seek not only My Ultimate Solution, Jesus—He can become whoever we need Him to be—but also the many solutions He has placed on this earth.

I wish I knew some of these concepts at an earlier age. I believe if I did, then my life may have unfolded a little differently. However, I am grateful for God's mercies which are new every day. I'm grateful for the opportunity to change.

I am hoping this book will prevent others from some of the poor choices I made, and at the same time lead others into a better way of life.

If you can have a relationship with our Great God, be stable mentally, have healthy relationships and a positive attitude, then you can live VICTORIOUSLY through any sickness or struggle you may face in your journey!

May our eyes be opened and remain open, to see what we need to see, to become who we need to be.

Thank you for reading and be blessed,

Angelena Cortello

"Angel"

angelcortello.com | angelenacortello@bellsouth.net

Helping Healing Hands

This book is a true miracle. I am eternally grateful to God for placing people in my path to be His healing hands and feet. Without their investment, I would not be the woman I am today and this book would not be possible. I want to thank God and all the people He used who helped make the dream He put in my heart happen.

First and foremost, I want to thank My Lord and Savior, Jesus Christ for delivering me from many unhealthy ways that were stopping me from living an abundant, productive life. For every personal failure or trying circumstance I face, He has been My Rock. Through trial and error, I have learned what needs to change in me. During times of personal frustration, I am grateful for His patience with me and for the determination He has placed inside my heart to continue moving forward on the path when it was not easy. I am looking forward to what He has for me as my journey continues.

Next, I would like to thank my family who has put up with me all these years and stood by me: Karen Gissin—You will always be "Momma." Steven Gissin—I always learn a lot when I listen to you talk. Frank and Cynthia Cortello—I admire the two of you's ability to press on even when life throws you a curve ball. Amanda—You have my heart and have since the first day I set eyes on you and got to hold you. I believe in You. Austin and Amelia—I cannot wait to see what God puts in you to do for Him in your future. To my grandparents, aunts, uncles and cousins—Our family Rocks and I love you all!!!!!

I would like to thank my friends who have taken the time to point me to The Ultimate Healer during different seasons of my path. I know I haven't always been easy to deal with, but thanks for being there: Sister Mickey Mangun, Nicole Brown, Mari Bobbitt, Pauni Abbott, Vani Marshall, Lin Signorelli, Michelle Bryant, Monica Wiggins, Cathy Mills, ms. Stephanie Frederic, Terri Eldrige (thanks for always keeping me laughing), Abigail Aycock (my partner in crime), Heather Freeman, Amber Delynn and Pamela Nolde.

I would like to thank those in my church family, those in the 12-Step community and those at CLASS (Central Louisiana AIDS Support Services) for being God's healing hands and feet during my journey.

I would like to thank Janae Borman and Cathy Holland who helped type up and edit some of the book.

I would like to thank Rebecca Boyett who spent countless hours helping me edit.

I would like to thank Brooke Davidson for the fabulous photo of me she made happen that is on the back cover of this book.

I would like to thank Naomi Tullos for trumping my idea of having an awareness ribbon on the cover that would represent as many emotional and physical issues as possible. She created the ribbon on the cover with words and we made sure each term matched the color of its awareness ribbon.

I would like to thank Heather Briley Bynog for writing Part Four, "Healing Habits for a Healthy You."

I would like to thank Stephanie Frederic and Greg Holsen at FGW Productions of Los Angeles, CA for the graphic design on the cover with the ribbon Naomi Tullos and I created.

I would like to thank Rachael Hartman and Our Written Lives for the formatting and layout of the book, and for publishing Healing Letters.

~Angel

Contents

Part One • 11

140 Days of Healing Letters to God

Part Two • 157

Health Awareness

Part Three • 167

Healing Scriptures

Part Four • 173

Healing Habits for a Healthy You

Healing Letters to God

Part One

> "The quality of a man's life is in direct proportion to his commitment to excellence, regardless of his chosen field of endeavor." Vince Lombardi

ALPHA,

Today I can and will begin again. It is high time to recommit some areas of my life to You and to the purpose You have called me to fulfill. You are the beginning. I want to begin again. Sometimes taking that first unknown step is the hardest leap of faith, but I have to start somewhere. Why not now? Why not with You? I refuse to allow myself to stick with what is unhealthy for me and familiar to me, out of fear of facing something new because it is uncomfortable or out of my comfort zone. When I face my fears, it builds my self-esteem. I can do anything with You in my life. I choose to make the first step with motivation and determination. The first step to changing for the better has to include You.

Love,
Your Child

Genesis 1:1 *"In the beginning God created the heaven and the earth."*

Romans 13:11-12 *"And that, knowing the time, that now it is high time to awake out of sleep: for now is our salvation nearer than when we believed. The night is far spent, the day is at hand: let us therefore cast off the works of darkness, and let us put on the armour of light."*

"Life is a great big canvas, and you should throw all the paint on it you can."
Danny Kaye

CREATOR,

Thank You, Lord, for loving me enough to create me in Your image and allow me to enjoy Your beautiful creation. Sometimes when I look out at nature, the beauty of it takes my breath away. No one but You could come up with these brilliant ideas in the creation of this world I get to live in. When I put myself or others down, let me be reminded I am putting down Your great work. We are the apple of Your eye. You are the greatest artist ever! Help me in this new season to always look for the good in every person and every situation as I move forward with You into everything You have for me to do.

Love,
Your Child

Genesis 1:27 *"So God created man in his own image; in the image of God created he him; male and female created he them."*

Genesis 1:31 *"And God saw everything that he had made, and, behold, it was very good. And the evening and the morning were the sixth day."*

"Idolatry is the practice of seeking the source and provision of what we need either physically or emotionally in someone or something other than the One True God. It is the tragically pathetic attempt to squeeze life out of lifeless forms that cannot help us meet our real needs." Scott J. Hafemann

SAVIOR,

Thank You for saving my life. Because of Your sacrifice for me, I have an opportunity to be with You forever and ever. Help me not to idolize people and put them in Your place. When I do that, I am let down because people cannot do what only You and Your power can do. People are a cheap substitute for You. People have the ability to let people down, but You never let me down. I will not give people the power to control my relationship with You. I will not use hypocrites as an excuse for why I am not where I need to be in You. I also do not want to put myself in Your place in my life. I do not want to live my life without You leading me, delivering me, healing me and saving me. It is Your power that I have to tap into daily to be able to fulfill Your purpose. I cannot do this alone. Thank You for saving me from myself.

Love, Your Child

Leviticus 19:4 *"Turn ye not unto idols, nor make to yourselves molten gods: I am the Lord Your God."*

John 3:16 *"For God so loved the world, that he gave His only begotten Son, that whosoever believeth in him should not perish, but have everlasting life."*

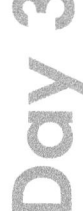

> "The optimist already sees the scar over the wound;
> the pessimist still sees the wound underneath the scar." Ernst Schroder

HEALER,

    I trust in Your Word. I trust You with the outcome of my life in spite of my circumstances. I know You are healing my heart, my mind and my body. You use many methods to fulfill Your purpose and work. You use doctors, medicine, counseling and support groups. You can work instantly through a simple prayer for a miracle or choose to work slowly through a process miracle. Either way You choose, it is still You! And either way, it is still a miracle! I will stay focused on the progress I am making each day in being a healthier person.

    When my heart is broken, You heal it. When my mind is broken, You heal it. When my body is broken, You heal it. Your life heals my life. Thank You for being beautifully broken so that I can be healed. Help me to recognize Your healing hands and accept the manner in which You choose to heal me.

Love, Your Child

Psalms 34:18 *"The Lord is nigh unto them that are of a broken heart; and saveth such as be of a contrite spirit."*

Psalms 147:3 *"He healeth the broken in heart, and bindeth up their wounds."*

> "I would like to be remembered as a person who wanted to be free . . . so other people would be also free." Rosa Parks

DELIVERER,

    I do not have to live a life where my unhealthy cravings are controlling me. What You did on the Cross of Calvary destroyed the power of sin in my life. You rose on the third day and conquered the power of death. That same Spirit lives inside of me. It is the strength that helps me to do the right thing when my sinful human nature wants to do the wrong thing. A friend once asked me: "What is the first thing that comes up in your mind as far as how to handle a difficult situation?" I told my friend how I wanted to incorrectly handle it out of my anger. My friend's response was, "You might want to do the opposite of that because the opposite is probably the right way to handle it." You have freed me of the power and control of sin over my life. I am no longer a slave to sin. I do not have to live by every impulsive feeling I get. Some of my feelings cannot be trusted. I have to do what You want. You have pulled me out of darkness and into Your marvelous light. My life is different and new because of it. Your Word teaches me what is right in Your eyes. This is why prayer and the reading of Your Word is so important. It feels good to be truly free from the things and people that I once allowed to control me before I truly experienced Your delivering power. Thank You. I don't ever want to live like that again. Show me how to maintain my deliverance.

Love,
Your Child

Psalms 18:2 "The Lord is my rock, and my fortress, and my deliverer; my God, my strength, in whom I will trust; my buckler, and the horn of my salvation, and my high tower."

"Him that I love, I wish to be free—even from me." Anne Morrow Lindbergh

FRIEND,

You are my best friend. You know everything about me and understand me better than anyone else. Help me to be friendly to others. I should want what is best for others and should desire to help them achieve their potential in living out their dreams. I should not be jealous or envious at their success. I should not try to find something wrong with their success. I should celebrate with them their success. Being a good friend, I should respect other people's space and allow people the freedom to make their own choices. I should respect the boundaries they create, whether I agree or disagree with them. I should not gossip about them or share their private matters with others. Help me to be a safe, trustworthy friend. I should love people so much that when it is time for them to leave my life to fulfill Your purpose elsewhere, I let them go with joy for their new season. I should not try to stop them. I should not try to hold them back to have them for myself. Also, help me to encourage people when they need it. When a friend falls down in any area of their life, let me be the friend who has the mercy and compassion to support them as they get back up. I do not want to be the one that makes it harder for them to start over or change. I do not want to remind them of their past failures because that can discourage them in their journey.

Love, Your Child

Proverbs 18:24 *"A man that hath friends must show himself friendly, and there is a friend that sticketh closer than a brother."*

"Love talked about can be easily turned aside, but love demonstrated is irresistible." W. Stanley Mooneyham

LOVER OF MY SOUL,

You loved me when I did not know how to love myself or anyone else. I did not even know what healthy love was, but now You are showing me. Love is enduring, patient, merciful, compassionate, truthful, and just. Love is not envious, controlling, self-seeking, boastful, arrogant, or rude. It believes everyone has potential. It builds people up and does not tear down. It loves righteousness and purity. It gives people the time they need to grow. It does not hold grudges, but forgives quickly. The inability to love and trust others can lead to isolation and depression. Fear of abandonment creates controlling and possessive people. True love is willing to let go of the need to be emotionally attached; it allows people to go in and out of our lives freely. It is free from the fear of rejection. Sometimes we outgrow people and sometimes people outgrow us; that is alright. Love is the ability to enjoy someone or something without needing it to survive emotionally because people will avoid me if the only reason they are in my life is to fulfill a selfish, emotional need. I want to love like You love. I know that my actions speak louder than anything I say. Help me to see people with Your eyes and not my own. Love is the most awesome and powerful force in the world. Let me example it correctly.

Love,
Your Child

1 John 4:8 "He that loveth not, knoweth not God, for God is love."

"Good mentors are essential for a successful career." Lailah Gifty Akita

COUNSELOR,

I can talk to You about anything. Constant complaining to others can result in toxic and even broken relationships, but You can handle hearing all of my concerns and understand where I am better than anyone else. Your Words in return are the best advice. You can guide me, and give me wisdom and insight to make certain decisions to bring about the expected end that You have for me. Help me to go to You first with my needs before talking to anyone else. I want You to be first in my life in everything and all of my decisions. Confirm Your will and Word for my life through my leaders when I talk to them. Help me to be open to the suggestions of the wise counsel that You place in my life and not defensive, but to consider it.

Love,
Your Child

Judges 18:5 "And they said unto him, Ask counsel, we pray thee, of God, that we may know whether our way which we go shall be prosperous."

Proverbs 19:2 "Hear counsel and receive instruction, that thou mayest be wise in thy latter end."

> "Temptation usually comes in through a door that has deliberately been left open." Arnold H. Glasow

REDEEMER,

Thank You for helping me recover from the damage my choices have caused. Your life released me from the debt of sin. When I strayed away from You and lived for the enemy of my soul, You reached out to me and brought me back to You. You paid the price that I should have paid. There are so many different times that I can look back on of when I know You were intervening in my behalf when I was not where I needed to be in You. Thank You for never giving up on trying to get my attention when I felt so stuck in darkness. You are my redeemer. You redeem the choices and words of my past that were not in accordance with Your will. Help me to give others the same opportunity to redeem themselves when they have done wrong to me. Thank You for taking me back when I did not deserve it. Help me to continue to live a redeemed life by showing me the triggers and doors of temptation that I have left open.

Love,
Your Child

Isaiah 43:11 "*But now thus said the Lord that created thee, O Jacob, and he that formed thee, O Israel, Fear not: for I have redeemed thee, I have called thee by thy name; thou art mine.*"

Galatians 4:3-6 "*Even so we, when we were children, were in bondage under the elements of the world: But when the fullness of the time was come, God sent forth his Son, made of a woman, made under the law, To redeem them that were under the law, that we might receive the adoption of sons. And because ye are sons, God hath sent forth the Spirit of his Son into your hearts, crying, Abba, Father.*"

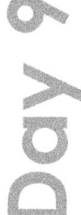

> "The pessimist complains about the wind; the optimist expects it to change; the realist adjusts the sails." William Arthur Ward

ENDING,

You are the beginning and the end at the same time. How do You do it? My brain struggles with fully understanding it. I do know this: some endings are necessary before new things can be birthed. Give me peace when You choose to end a season or end any relationship in my life. Sometimes You have to move things or people out of the way before new things and new people can come into my life. Help me to adjust to the changes You are making in my life. Help me to accept Your will and Your timing when people, jobs, health or any circumstances change and a season ends.

Love,
Your Child

Revelation 1:8 *"I am Alpha and Omega, the beginning and the ending, said the Lord, which is, and which was, and which is to come, the Almighty."*

"To be successful you must accept all challenges that come your way. You can't just accept the ones you like." Mike Gafka

NEW,

Every day I wake up with a new day, full of new choices, new challenges, new adventures and a new opportunity. I choose to let go of the past and walk in a new path of righteousness. I am a new creature in You because I have been baptized in Your name. Therefore, I want to live this new day, keeping in mind that I am a Christian. Renew my mind daily and help me to be Christlike in my attitude, character, words and choices.

Love,
Your Child

2 Corinthians 5:17 *"Therefore if any man be in Christ, he is a new creature: old things are passed away; behold, all things are become new."*

Galatians 3:27 *"For as many of you as have been baptized into Christ have put on Christ.'*

Ephesians 4:23-24 *"And be renewed in the spirit of your mind; And that ye put on the new man which after God is created in righteousness and true holiness."*

> "Self-respect is the fruit of discipline; the sense of dignity grows with the ability to say no to oneself." Abraham Joshva Heschel

THE ONE WHO DENIES HIMSELF,

Help me to be reminded that self-will and Your will are two totally different things. My self-will or flesh wants to do the wrong thing at times. I have to do what I know is right, not live by my emotions and do everything I feel like doing. I choose to be led by You and what is right. I will not allow my emotions to make my decisions. My life is meant to be lived for Your glory and purpose to be fulfilled. Give me Your vision for my life, and show me the steps I need to take to fulfill it. I don't want my ways, will or agenda. I want Your ways, will and agenda.

Love,
Your Child

Matthew 16:24 *"Then said Jesus unto his disciples, If any man will come after me, let him deny himself, and take up his cross, and follow me."*

> "The most important thing in communication is to hear what isn't being said."
> Peter F. Drucker

HEARER,

I cannot thank You enough for always being there for me and hearing what I have to say. You are available at any time, day or night. I want to hear You, to hear what You have to say to me and to this world we live in. I want to know Your thoughts, Your feelings and Your heartbeat. I want to look for You all throughout my day and try to hear what You are saying. I like hearing You through a sunset, music, and other people. My favorite is when I hear You while reading Your Word. I do not want to just hear You every now and then. I will position myself to hear You more. I will do what You are telling me to do, and be obedient to Your Word and will. Let me be attentive when listening to others. Help me to discern the motive behind what they are saying. Let me see the situation through their perspective. I do not want to act as if my experiences are the same as others. This can come across as insensitive and self-centered. I want people to know that I care about what they have to say. Let me keep eye contact. I will put my phone down. I do not want to be easily distracted by what is going on around me. I know I want people's undivided attention when talking to them; let me do the same for others.

Love, Your Child

Psalms 121:4 *"Behold, he that keepeth Israel shall neither slumber nor sleep."*

James 1:22 *"But be ye doers of the word, and not hearers only, deceiving your own selves."*

> "It is far more impressive when others discover your good qualities without your help." Judith S. Martin

EXALTED ONE,

You are amazing! You deserve to be exalted and lifted up every day! I honor You. May everyone and everything exalt You! Help my attitude when I find myself boasting or exalting myself instead of You. I do not want to have an attitude of arrogance and thinking I am better than everyone else. Help me to not get a "big head" when I am Blessed with a great accomplishment. I want to give You the credit, not myself. I do not want to feel more important than I am. I will not say things fishing for a compliment. Life should not be lived for recognition. I will do my best and as much as I can because it is the right thing to do, not for the praise of people which belongs to You, or to create the reaction I want. Doing what is right is good enough for me. I want to remain humble even when I am blessed with success. I know I am not "all that." You are "all that." I love You.

Love, Your Child

Psalms 57:11 *"Be thou exalted, O God, above the heavens: let thy glory be above all the earth."*

Proverbs 16:18 *"Pride goeth before destruction, and an haughty spirit before a fall."*

Luke 18:14 *"I tell you, this man went down to his house justified rather than the other: for every one that exalted himself shall be abased; and he that humbleth himself shall be exalted."*

"Prayer is when you talk to God; meditation is when you listen to God."
Diana Robinson

FOUNTAIN,

You are my ultimate source—out of You I find everything I need. Even if my mind or body is failing me, You become whoever and whatever I need. I cannot live my life fully if I am spiritually empty. Can You show me the different ways that You want to fill me up? Daily I will draw my strength from You by spending time with You in prayer and in Your Word, so that I have what is needed to face the obstacles of the day. I know I need You to be able to live this life. Quitting is unacceptable. I can get through the day because I have You.

Love,
Your Child

Psalms 36:9 *"For with Thee is the fountain of life; in Thy light shall we see light."*

"Being considerate of others will take you further in life than a college degree." Marian Wright Edelman

CONSIDERATE ONE,

Thank You for always being considerate of my feelings and what is best for me. Like You, help me also to be considerate of other people's feelings throughout the day. Let me be genuinely concerned about the happiness of others. You know how to draw the best out of me. When You intervene unexpectedly, I will welcome Your sweet surprises. I will trust Your divine interruptions in my life, even physical infirmities and afflictions. Sometimes You slow me down for a reason. I will allow Your plan for me to unfold as You wish, whether I agree or disagree with it. I will embrace the changes involved in Your will for my journey.

Love,
Your Child

Hebrews 4:15 *For we have not an high priest which cannot be touched with the feelings of our infirmities; but was in all points tempted like as we are, yet without sin."*

> "Art doesn't reproduce the visible but rather makes it visible." Paul Klee

LIGHT,

    I always feel a dark, bad feeling when doing something I know I am not supposed to be doing. I do not want to live in darkness. Your light reveals the darkness in my life and heart so that I have an opportunity to choose to stop living with dark, evil ways. Reveal any and all darkness in my life and rid my life of it. Your light feels so much better and right. I choose to live in the light of what is right. My life cannot shine unless Your light is in me and shining through me. Let Your light shine through me, revealing the truth and lies that I believe about myself. Set me free from faulty thinking about myself. Belief includes action. I believe what Your Word says about me. My actions will reveal my beliefs. Help me to portray what You and Your Word stands for.

    Love,
    Your Child

John 12:46 *"I am come a light into the world, that whosoever believeth on me should not abide in darkness."*

"And almost every one when age, disease, or sorrow strike him, inclines to think there is a God, or something very like Him." Arthur Hugh Clough

MYSTERY,

I do not want to only seek You when in desperate times. I want to seek You at all times. I found something so real that I cannot walk away. I cannot fully explain You, but I do not have to in order to know that You are real. If I knew everything about You, then why would I need faith? You are a true mystery unfolding; one that I get a little understanding of as each day of my journey unfolds. I love it! It keeps me spiritually hungry and wanting to know You more. You are very intriguing! I know enough and I cannot wait until we meet face to face, and more of Your mystery will be revealed.

Love,
Your Child

Ephesians 6:19 *"And for me that utterance may be given unto me, that I may open my mouth boldly, to make known the mystery of the gospel."*

"And almost every one when age, disease, or sorrow strike him, inclines to think there is a God, or something very like Him." Arthur Hugh Clough

Mystery,

I do not want to only seek You when in desperate times. I want to seek You at all times. I found something so real that I cannot walk away. I cannot fully explain You, but I do not have to in order to know that You are real. If I knew everything about You, then why would I need faith? You are a true mystery unfolding; one that I get a little understanding of as each day of my journey unfolds. I love it! It keeps me spiritually hungry and wanting to know You more. You are very intriguing! I know enough and I cannot wait until we meet face to face, and more of Your mystery will be revealed.

Love,
Your Child

Ephesians 6:19 *"And for me that utterance may be given unto me, that I may open my mouth boldly, to make known the mystery of the gospel."*

> "Art doesn't reproduce the visible but rather makes it visible." Paul Klee

LIGHT,

I always feel a dark, bad feeling when doing something I know I am not supposed to be doing. I do not want to live in darkness. Your light reveals the darkness in my life and heart so that I have an opportunity to choose to stop living with dark, evil ways. Reveal any and all darkness in my life and rid my life of it. Your light feels so much better and right. I choose to live in the light of what is right. My life cannot shine unless Your light is in me and shining through me. Let Your light shine through me, revealing the truth and lies that I believe about myself. Set me free from faulty thinking about myself. Belief includes action. I believe what Your Word says about me. My actions will reveal my beliefs. Help me to portray what You and Your Word stands for.

Love,
Your Child

John 12:46 *"I am come a light into the world, that whosoever believeth on me should not abide in darkness."*

"Criticism, like rain, should be gentle enough to nourish a man's growth without destroying his roots." Frank A. Clark

SPEAKER,

Thank You for everything You have spoken to me. I cherish every time we talk. Thank You for speaking to me at my level and in a way that You know I would understand. As the church is the Bride of Christ—with members all over the world as part of the body—let us all work together for Your kingdom's good and growth. When I speak of You, let it be with boldness, clarity and anointing. I love it when I get to feel Your presence and Your power when I am speaking of You. It is a privilege anytime I get to talk about the One I love the most! When speaking to others in front of a group for any reason, let me be dressed nicely—representing You well. Let me bring humor to the crowd. Let me know my topic well. Let me be easily understood and not too wordy. Let me not be driven by the opinions of others. I will not allow the fear of failure to stop me from speaking. As Your spokesperson, let me always speak with the proper balance of truth and grace. Help me to see the best in others, to accept constructive criticism, and be open to the ideas of others. Help me to show mercy toward others when they fall. Bless me as I do my best to be a blessing to You. Thank You for every opportunity where I get to be Your spokesperson—speaking of Your great love, mercy and ways!

Love, Your Child

Ephesians 4:15-16 *"But speaking the truth in love, may grow up into him in all things, which is the head, even Christ: From whom the whole body fitly joined together and compacted by that which every joint supplieth, according to the effectual working in the measure of every part, maketh increase of the body unto the edifying of itself in love."*

> "The most powerful weapon on earth is the human soul on fire."
> **Ferdinand Foch**

GOLD,

Lord, help me to realize that You have me in the process of sanctification. In that process, You are refining me in the fire of trials and tests so that I may be pure as gold and more effective for Your glory. The fire of Your Spirit burns away the impurities in me. You reveal what needs to change in me through failures in relationships, jobs and unhealthy choices. Stress is the outward manifestation that reveals what is going on inside of us. Stress can destroy my physical health. I will remove any unnecessary stressors in my life so that I can stay as healthy as I can. Help me to not be a victim of my emotions or a victim of my circumstances. I do not want a victim mentality. I want a victor mentality. With Your help, I will responsibly deal with what is revealed to me about myself as You open my eyes and enlighten me. Take away all desire for sin and impurities. Let my life bring You glory as I dwell in Your glorious presence.

Love, Your Child

Zechariah 13:9 *"And I will bring the third part through the fire, and will refine them as silver is refined, and will try them as gold is tried: they shall call on my name, and I will hear them: I will say, It is my people: and they shall say, The Lord is my God."*

Matthew 3:11 *"I indeed baptize you with water unto repentance: but he that cometh after me is mightier than I whose shoes I am not worthy to bear: he shall baptize you with the Holy Ghost, and with fire."*

"Morality is its own advocate; it is never necessary to apologize for it."
Edith L. Harrell

RENEWER,

I do not want to live by this world's standard. I want to live by Your standard. One of Your gifts to us is Your Word. I learn what Your standard is by reading Your Word. I learn what is right and what is wrong in Your eyes when I read Your Word. Your Word cleanses my mind and teaches me how to think. Help me to not be easily influenced by the opinions of others and the pressures of this world that go against what You are speaking to my heart. Let me not try to change Your Word to fit my lifestyle and desires. Let my mind and life be conformed to Your Word and Your will.

Love,
Your Child

Romans 12:2 *"And be not conformed to this world: but be ye transformed by the renewing of your mind, that ye may prove what is that good, and acceptable, and perfect, will of God."*

> "Most of us ask for advice when we know the answer but want a different one." Ivern Ball

ANSWER,

    Life has created a lot of questions in my mind. You are the Ultimate Answer. I may not have all of the answers, and that is okay. I do not have to anymore. I no longer live my life, trying to figure it all out. I have made peace with having no answers to all of my questions. Sometimes Your answers are not immediate. Help me to accept Your divine delays. When I come into Your presence in prayer, I get to share with You my most intimate and secret thoughts. It is then I realize that I am with "The Answer" that is going to get me through this life. That is enough for me. Being with You, Jesus, is enough to satisfy my unanswered questions.

Love,
Your Child

Psalms 118:5 *"I called upon the Lord in distress: the Lord answered me, and set me in a large place."*

> "Correction does much, but encouragement does more."
> Johann Wolfgang von Goethe

ENCOURAGER,

You encourage me every day. When the bird outside the window sings a sweet hymn early in the morning, I know is You encouraging me to start my day. When I receive an unexpected blessing given to me through one of Your children, I know it is You encouraging me along my journey. When I feel Your Spirit while worshiping with other believers in church on Sunday morning, I know it is You lifting me up. The way You flirt with me throughout the day, I know it is You who is my True Love. Help me to be an encourager, too. Help me to motivate and encourage myself and others. Encouragers always make people feel better and believe their dreams are possible. My encouraging words and actions paint a canvas of my day. What painting am I creating? How important do people feel when they leave my presence? I want them to feel loved and encouraged. At the same time, help me to acknowledge the various ways others give me love and encouragement because I do not want them to feel unappreciated or taken for granted. Guard my tongue from complaining, gossip and negativity and let my words only lift up and encourage others. Bless my spirit with gratitude for all the ways You encourage me. Let me be an instrument of encouragement to others for You; that is one of the ways I get to blow kisses back at You.

Love, Your Child

1 Samuel 30:6 *"And David was greatly distressed; for the people spake of stoning him, because the soul of all the people was grieved, every man for his sons and for his daughters: but David encouraged himself in the Lord his God."*

"One of the secrets of a long and fruitful life is to forgive everybody, everything, every night before you go to bed." Ann Landers

LONG LIFE,

    I will pick and choose my battles because not everything is worth fighting over. I choose to let things go that are unimportant for me to be upset about. We all make mistakes and deserve mercy and compassion. Life is too short to focus on things that do not matter in the long run. Help me to stay focused on the "big picture." Every day is a new day that I want filled with love. My life on this earth is only temporal. Help me to take care of the body that You gave me so that I can live on this earth as long as I am needed to fulfill my purpose here. Because I am saved and choose to live for You, regardless of how long I have on this earth, I will have eternal life with You. I will live a productive life as a Godly citizen of society until I spend forever with You, the lover of my soul.

Love,
Your Child

Psalms 91:6 *"With long life, will I satisfy him, and shew him my salvation."*

> "The hardest arithmetic to master is that which enables us to count our blessings." Eric Hoffer

REJOICE,

    Help me to keep an attitude of gratitude and rejoice in You. Every challenge I face is an opportunity where You get to be glorified in a greater way through me. Self-pity is counterproductive and only makes me feel worse. When I am stuck in self-pity, remind me to stop and make a list of all of the blessings in my life so that I can get myself back in focus. I want to rejoice in You more. When I feel the hard knocks of life, remind me that my physical and emotional sufferings will not last forever because "joy cometh in the morning". If my "morning" does not arrive during my time on earth, then I know it will definitely come when I am in eternity with You. When I feel like my life is the greatest, I know there is always someone better off than me; therefore, I will stay balanced because my life was meant for me. I will not compare my life to others. Other people's lives with their triumphs and tragedies were meant for them. I am happy because I get to live my days out with You in them. I will rejoice with the life You have given me.

    Love,
    Your Child

Psalms 30:5 "… weeping may endure for a night, but joy cometh in the morning."

Psalms 70:4 "Let all those that seek thee rejoice and be glad in thee: and let such as love thy salvation say continually, let God be magnified."

Day 25

> "Self-discipline is when your conscience tells you to do something and you don't talk back." W.K. Hope

SOFT ANSWER,

    You are all about peace and keeping the peace. When someone upsets me, I have the tendency to want to lash out at them in anger, but that is like pouring gasoline on a fire. It adds fuel to a fire that is already there. I do not want to respond in a way that can make the situation worse. When I am angry at someone, with Your help I will look at them through Your eyes of love. If I feel someone is wrong but I know they do not believe they are, help me to accept that their perception is their reality. I can accept them as "human," like me. I will choose to forgive because forgiveness is one of the highest manifestations of Your love. After all, if I expect people to be merciful toward me when I fall, then I need to be able to show everyone else the same respect. I want to pour water on the fire and put it out. Help me to respond with a soft answer. If I cannot do that, give me the desire to count to ten in my head, take a deep breath, consider the "big picture," and respond softly. Put angels in front of my tongue.

    Love,
    Your Child

Proverbs 15:1 *"A soft answer turneth away wrath: but grievous words stir up anger."*

> "There is nothing like sealing a letter to inspire a fresh thought." Al Bernstein

PROPHET,

It is amazing to me how the scriptures confirm themselves. Even though there are many writers of the Bible, I know the Holy Ghost, Your spirit, is who guided all of the prophets to write about You and to give us instructions for healthy living. The Bible is divinely inspired by Your spirit. I want to know the truth about You and about life. Therefore, as You guide me in my journey, I will seek Your Word and watch Your truths transform my life. Thank You for Your wonderful Words!

Love,
Your Child

2 Peter 1:21 *"For the prophecy came not in the old time by the will of men: but holy men of God spake as they were moved by the Holy Ghost."*

> "No one is useless in this world who lightens the burden of it for anyone else."
> Charles Dickens

WARMTH,

When I see someone with a need that I am able to meet, help me to meet it. If it is winter time and I see a homeless person on a corner who is cold, let me give them a blanket. It does no good for me to believe in helping others, if I do not act on my beliefs and actually reach out to them. I want to be Your hands and feet. I want to provide when I can. I will not give with any expectation of getting anything back. Love does for others without expectation and without using "giving" as a method of control. I will give out of love as You lead me. I will give simply because it is the right thing to do. You are my warmth; I want to be warmth for others who need it.

Love,
Your Child

James 2:15-17 *"If a brother or sister be naked, and destitute of daily food, And one of you say unto them, Depart in peace, be ye warmed and filled; notwithstanding ye give them not those things which are needful to the body; what doth it profit? Even so faith, if it hath not works, is dead, being alone."*

"It is a perplexing and unpleasant truth that when men have something worth fighting for, they do not feel like fighting." Eric Hoffer

WEAPON AGAINST THE ENEMY,

Your Word, Your truth, Your blood and Your name are my greatest weapons in the spirit realm. Let me be reminded that I am not fighting against people. I am fighting against the sin that is controlling people to try to destroy Your will. Therefore, I pray against the evil spirits and sin that are trying to keep people bound and enslaved to an evil world of darkness. The enemy uses faulty thinking and belief systems that are contrary to Your Word; when this happens, I will refocus on the truth. I will correct my misconceptions. If I get out of focus, I pray the healthy people in my path will remind me of the truth. I choose to say "no" to sin and to say "yes" to You and Your righteous ways! I do not know why I choose to do wrong sometimes, but I will not give up in my attempt to obtain the victory. When I fall, I will forgive myself as You have forgiven me, and I will move on. I will not allow others to put me on a guilt trip over something I corrected and prayed about. I will fight for others to make it, and I will fight to do right until my journey ends.

Love,
Your Child

2 Corinthians 10:3-6 *"For though we walk in the flesh, we do not war after the flesh: (For the weapons of our warfare are not carnal, but mighty through God to the pulling down of strong holds;) casting down imaginations, and every high thing that exalteth itself against the knowledge of God, and bringing into captivity every thought to the obedience of Christ; And having in a readiness to revenge all disobedience, when your obedience is fulfilled."*

"Trust in God and do something." Mary Lyon

I Am,

You are exactly what I need to get through this life. You never said I would not struggle with sin, sickness, poverty or relationships. However, You are who is going to be with me through this life and who helps me get through this life. You also give me the strength I need to live with the consequences of my choices. I will not blame my past, my family or unfair circumstances for the wrong choices I make as an adult. The "blame game" removes the responsibility for my choices that rightfully belongs to me. Blame is nothing but a victim mentality, an excuse to not change my ways and an avenue to gain pity from others. I will not allow my consequences or circumstances to become an excuse to be bitter, have self-pity, have self-hatred, harbor unforgiveness or have a negative attitude with You. I will accept responsibility for my part in every situation I am in. Because the One who created all things and died for me is on my side, I can make it. What better partner to have with me through this journey than the One who created the sun, moon, planets and all people? I can make it because I have You!

Love,
Your Child

Day 30

Exodus 3:13-15 *"And Moses said unto God, Behold, when I come unto the children of Israel, and shall say unto them, The God of your fathers hath sent me unto you; and they shall say to me, What is his name? What shall I say unto them? And God said unto Moses, I AM THAT I AM: and he said, Thus shalt thou say unto the children of Israel, I AM hath sent me unto you. And God said moreover unto Moses, Thus shalt thou say unto the children of Israel, The Lord God of your fathers, the God of Abraham, the God of Isaac, and the God of Jacob, hath sent me unto you: this is my name for ever, and this is my memorial unto all generations."*

> "In prayer it is better to have a heart without words than words without a heart." John Bunyan

INTERCESSOR,

Thank You for interceding and praying for me. Your Spirit prays through me when I am speaking in tongues, in that Heavenly language. Praying and interceding in tongues helps my infirmities. When I feel led to pray that way, I will. Interceding in tongues also prays Your will into existence. When I am interceding, I am standing in the gap spiritually for others. I am praying for You to intervene into their situation or need. I seek Your mercy in people's lives. I seek Your favor. Raise up more intercessors to pray for our world, our nation, those who are sick, those who are bound, and those struggling financially. Give me a burden to intercede for others in prayer—for their salvation, healing, deliverance and direction. Praying for others takes the focus off my own issues. At the same time, put me on someone's heart as they pray when I am going through something; I know we all need each other.

Love,
Your Child

Romans 8:26-28 *"Likewise the Spirit also helpeth our infirmities: for we know not what we should pray for as we ought: but the spirit itself maketh intercession for us with groanings which cannot be uttered. And he that searcheth the hearts knoweth what is the mind of the Spirit, because he maketh intercession for the saints according to the will of God. And we know that all things work together for good to them that love God, to them who are the called according to his purpose."*

"Lack of something to feel important about is almost the greatest tragedy a man may have." Arthur E. Morgan

MAJESTY,

You and Your mighty works are quite impressive. You are great, and everything that You have created is great. You have the victory over all sin and evil. You are in charge of everything. Everything was made by You and for You. Everything belongs to You, including me; I am Your child, Your creation. I am made in Your image, and I belong to You. I do not have to prove my worth to others by showing what I can afford to buy, by my level of success or position or by exaggerating the truth. Exaggerations are really lies. I do not have to get my value from how much I am recognized or from the applause of people. None of these things can truly validate me. Only You validate me. I know You love me, or You would not have created me and died to save me. I am not defined by the opinion of others. I am not even defined by my own opinion of myself. I am defined by Your opinion of me. I am Your child. Therefore, I am royalty. I deserve to be treated the best, by both myself and others. At the same time, I will treat others with respect because, as Your creation, they too have value.

Love,
Your Child

1 Chronicles 29:11 *"Thine, O Lord, is the greatness, and the power, and the glory, and the victory, and the majesty: for all that is in the heaven and in the earth is thine; thine is the kingdom, O Lord, and thou art exalted as head above all."*

Revelation 4:11 *"Thou art worthy, O Lord, to receive glory and honour and power: for thou hast created all things, and for thy pleasure they are and were created."*

"A master can tell you what he expects of you. A teacher, though, awakens your own expectations." Patricia Neal with Richard DeNeut

RABBI,

You are my leader. You are my teacher. I submit my thoughts, words and actions today to Your will and leadership. I put You in the driver's seat. You are the pilot. I trust wherever You lead me, and I trust in whatever You want to teach me today. Before making any decisions, I will bring it to You in prayer and fasting. I will research and look into all the facts, making a list of the pros and cons. Also, any leaders that You have placed in my path—teachers, bosses, parents, and mentors—I will respect them and submit to their authority over my life. Throughout this process, You are helping me to make an informed decision.

Love,
Your Child

John 3:2 *"The same came to Jesus by night, and said unto him, Rabbi, we know that thou art a teacher come from God: for no man can do these miracles that thou doest, except God be with him."*

Hebrews 13:17 *"Obey them that have the rule over you, and submit yourselves: for they watch for your souls, as they that must give account, that they may do it with joy, and not with grief: for that is unprofitable for you."*

> "Self-pity in its early stages is as snug as a feather mattress. Only when it hardens does it become uncomfortable." Maya Angelou

DAY STAR,

    Let Your light shine through all of my gloomy days. I will look for Your light in my darkest of days and nights. I will focus on what is going right in my life. I will not feel sorry for myself because I know that self-pity leads to self-destructive choices, which results in further depression. Self-pity is a form of pride that keeps the focus on myself in a negative way. Self-pity can also stop me from being proactive while living in the present moment. It is a time waster. It is full of useless excuses. It leads to me comparing myself with others, which is pointless because Your plan is different, unique and tailor made for me. Self-pity depletes our desire to move forward. It is a killer of motivation and a killer of joy. So, I will look to You, Day Star, and choose to let Your light shine on me and through me to pierce the darkness around me and in me.

Love,
Your Child

2 Peter 1:19 "*We have also a more sure word of prophecy; where unto ye do well that ye take heed, as unto a light that shineth in a dark place, until the day dawn, and the day star arise in your hearts . . .*"

"The road to success is dotted with many tempting parking spaces." Will Rogers

THE ONE I CRAVE,

    The truth is, at times I enjoy being in the flesh or sinning. However, I know it does not please You. Change the desires and cravings of my heart. Help me to hate what You hate and love what You love. Changing my heart's cravings is something only You can do. Let my desires line up with Your will.

    I know that it is not Your will for me to skip my medications. I know it is not Your will for me to overeat or to eat what I know I should not have. I know it is not Your will for me to be in an abusive relationship. I know it is not Your will for me to chase the person that You do not want me to have. I know it is not Your will for me to neglect my health. I know it is not Your will for me to put illegal substances into my body.

    I know it is not Your will for me to practice revenge. I know it is not Your will for me to destroy other people's reputations. I know it is not Your will for me to be jealous. I know it is not Your will for me to feel sorry for myself. I know it is not Your will for me to have a negative outlook on life.

I know it is not Your will for me to be unreliable in my commitments. Giving in to unhealthy temptations and cravings is an unnecessary detour off the journey that You have me on. Help me to stay on Your chosen path.

Love,
Your Child

Job 21:14 *"Therefore they say unto God, Depart from us; for we desire not the knowledge of thy ways."*

Psalms 37:4-5 *"Delight thyself also in the Lord; and he shall give thee the desires of thine heart.*

Commit thy way unto the Lord; trust also in him; and he shall bring it to pass."

Galatians 4:9 *"But now, after that ye have known God, or rather are known of God, how turn ye again to the week and beggarly elements, where unto ye desire again to be in bondage?"*

Ephesians 2:3-5 *"Among whom also we all had our conservation in times past in the lusts of our flesh, fulfilling the desires of the flesh and of the mind; and were by nature the children of wrath, even as others. But God, who is rich in mercy, for his great love wherewith he loved us, Even when we were dead in sins, hath quickened us together with Christ, (by grace ye are saved)"*

James 4:7 *"Submit yourselves therefore to God. Resist the devil, and he will flee from you."*

"Dreams and dedication are a powerful combination." William Longgood

DREAM COME TRUE,

    I used to think I knew what was best for me and that my ways and plans were better than Yours. When my agenda fell through and I let go of my idea of what I thought You had for my life, I discovered pieces of Your dream for my life that You wanted fulfilled. When I began to focus on making Your dreams come true, it was actually more satisfying than my plans could ever have been. Thank You for unfolding Your plan for my life. Thank You for letting me be a part of Your dream! I am honored to be Your dream come true.

    Love,
    Your Child

Isaiah 55:9 *"For as the heavens are higher than the earth, so are my ways higher than your ways, and my thoughts than your thoughts."*

Jeremiah 29:11 *"For I know the thoughts that I think toward you, saith the Lord, thoughts of peace, and not of evil, to give you an expected end."*

"The time to relax is when you don't have time for it." Sydney J. Harris

REST,

You are my resting place. Sometimes You call me to break away from everything and rest in Your presence. I do not have to feel guilty when I need a break to rest from work or helping others. If I do not have balance in my life and rest when it is time to rest, then I cannot be who I need to be for others or Your kingdom. Sleep deprivation causes accidents, affects job performance, and causes moodiness and irritability. It affects my focus, and it affects my memory. It also puts a strain on my physical health. When I rest, I am being restored and strengthened to fulfill Your work when my time of resting is up.

Love,
Your Child

Genesis 2:2 *"And on the seventh day God ended his work which he had made; and he rested on the seventh day from all his work which he had made."*

"Another flaw in the human character is that everyone wants to build and nobody wants to do maintenance." Kurt Vonnegut

CLEAN ONE,

Cleanse my mind and spirit with Your Word. Show me what to get rid of in my home or life that could be polluting my walk with You and my effectiveness in doing Your work. Is it certain music, films, or books? Is my social circle drawing me toward You and Your will or away from You? If it is not healthy or wholesome and is polluting my life, then give me the desire to strip it from my life. Help me to not be desensitized to sin, but to be more sensitive to what is good. Help me be more sensitive to You.

Love,
Your Child

2 Corinthians 7:1 *"Having therefore these promises, dearly beloved, let us cleanse ourselves from all filthiness of the flesh and spirit, perfecting holiness in the fear of God."*

"More important than a work of art itself is what it will sow. Art can die, a painting can disappear. What counts is the seed." Joan Miro

COMFORTER,

Your Spirit comforts me when I am grieving. There is no time table for how long it takes to grieve the loss of anyone or anything, including the loss of my health. Grief comes and goes. We are all different and grieve differently. It is not right to make anyone feel like there is a certain time to stop grieving. Whenever I am done grieving over one thing, there will always be something else to grieve over because life is constantly changing. With change, there are both losses and gains. I do not have to be afraid of feeling pain. The truth is, I can survive in spite of pain. I need to be patient with people who are grieving and pray for them and listen to them, as You do me. Help me to comfort others the way I would want to be comforted.

Love,
Your Child

John 14:26 "But the Comforter, which is the Holy Ghost, whom the Father will send in my name, he shall teach you all things, and bring all things to your remembrance, whatsoever I have said unto you."

John 16:7 "Nevertheless I tell you the truth; It is expedient for you that I go away: for if I go not away, the comforter will not come unto you; but if I depart, I will send him unto you.

"Half our life is spent trying to find something to do with the time we have rushed through life trying to save." Will Rogers

BALANCE,

    I know You want me to be balanced in all areas of my life. When I get off kilter, please help me to get my balance back. Help me balance my time and priorities — everything from family time, involvement in the community or church, housecleaning, exercise, doctor's appointments and eating right. Let me covet my time of prayer and meditation with You and in Your Word, keeping them first and foremost in my life. It is not good for me to spend all of my time on one thing to the exclusion of all others. It is important and necessary to balance my time amongst all of my responsibilities.

Love,
Your Child

Proverbs 11:1 *"A false balance is abomination to the Lord: but a just weight is his delight."*

> "One of the greatest sources of energy is pride in what you are doing."
>
> Spokes

ENERGY,

I love my life, and I love what I do. My calling on this earth motivates me to make a difference with the gift of life that each day brings. You are the life force who strengthens me to do what I need to do throughout my day. When I am weak, You become my energy to do what I need to do. To boost the energy You give me, You provided certain foods to help me on my way. I can eat almonds, dark chocolate, spinach, eggs and whole grains. I can take certain vitamins too such as B12 and iron. Thank You for providing on this Earth what I need to sustain my energy when feeling weak. I love the way You have provided everything I need in so many different ways.

Love,
Your Child

Psalms 18:1 *"I will love thee, O Lord, my strength."*

> "Everything should be made as simple as possible, but not simpler."
> — Albert Einstein

YOKE IS EASY,

Your "yoke" or "teachings" are always easier than what they seem. When I follow Your ways and teachings, I have peace because I know I am giving life my best shot and am seeking to please You. I do not have that same peace when willfully sinning. I feel condemned, convicted, guilty and dark when not doing what I am supposed to do. Your yoke is easy and makes me feel better. Your ways bring peace and abundant living. Thank You for keeping it easy and simple for all of us.

Love,
Your Child

Matthew 11:30 *"For my yoke is easy, and my burden is light."*

John 10:10 *"The thief cometh not, but for to steal, and to kill, and to destroy: I am come that they might have life, and that they might have it more abundantly."*

> "You can measure a man by the opposition it takes to discourage him."
>
> Robert C. Savage

SOBRIETY,

Help me to not give in to anything excessively. Help me to stay balanced and practice self-control daily. Let me be aware of the schemes the enemy will try to use to get me off track in order to destroy my consistency and balance. When under pressure or dealing with any setbacks or resistance to doing the right thing, I will stay on the course You have set for me. I will not be easily influenced or tossed about from my foundation by ways that are not of You. I cannot control every thought that goes through my head, but I can control how long I dwell on it. Therefore, I choose to not dwell on toxic thoughts that can lead to self-destructive habits. I know You want me to be healthy, happy and productive. I know the enemy will try to use misunderstandings, unfair circumstances, personality conflicts and my personal failures to make me stumble, but my mind is made up. I will not allow these things to stop me from being used by You. The enemy will not win, and I will overcome all of it with Your grace.

Love, Your Child

1 Peter 5:8 *"Be sober, be vigilant; because your adversary the devil, as a roaring lion, walketh about, seeking whom he may devour."*

Ephesians 4: 14-15 *"That we henceforth be no more children, tossed to and fro, and carried about with every wind of doctrine, by the sleight of men, and cunning craftiness, whereby they lie in wait to deceive; But speaking the truth in love, may grow up into him in all things, which is the head, even Christ."*

> "We learn to walk by stumbling." Bulgarian Proverb

EXPERIENCE,

    People can have their opinions and criticize my faith in You; however, no one can take away my very personal and private experiences with You during times where You have made Yourself very obvious and real to me. Thank You for all the times I have experienced You in special ways in my life. Also, I have found my experiences in life have been my greatest teachers of true wisdom and insight. I am not afraid to fall down every now and then because I know failures are only opportunities to learn and grow. You are more concerned with my character and growth than my comfort. Thank You for the good and the bad experiences that have taught me what I needed to learn to be a healthier me. I will intentionally follow Your course for my life.

Love,
Your Child

Ecclesiastes 1:16 *"I communed with mine own heart, saying, Lo, I am come to great estate, and have gotten more wisdom than all they that have been before me in Jerusalem: yea, my heart had great experience of wisdom and knowledge."*

"The miracle is this—the more we share, the more we have." Leonard Nimoy

OFFERING,

Jesus, You are the ultimate offering of life for life. Whenever I give an offering, let it not be something I feel that I have to do. An offering is something I want to do to bless Your kingdom and its people. I can give to missionary work. I can also bless someone financially who I know is struggling. One thing I have learned is I cannot out-give You. You will always return the favor in some form and at just the right time. Thank You for that. I want to give selflessly like You.

Love,
Your Child

Genesis 22:8 *"And Abraham said, My son, God will provide himself a lamb for a burnt offering: so they went both of them together."*

Ezekiel 46:13 *"Thou shalt daily prepare a burnt offering unto the Lord of a lamb of the first year without blemish: thou shalt prepare it every morning."*

John 1:29 *"The next day John seeth Jesus coming unto him, and saith, Behold the Lamb of God, which taketh away the sin of the world."*

"The miracle is this—the more we share, the more we have." Leonard Nimoy

OFFERING,

Jesus, You are the ultimate offering of life for life. Whenever I give an offering, let it not be something I feel that I have to do. An offering is something I want to do to bless Your kingdom and its people. I can give to missionary work. I can also bless someone financially who I know is struggling. One thing I have learned is I cannot out-give You. You will always return the favor in some form and at just the right time. Thank You for that. I want to give selflessly like You.

Love,
Your Child

Genesis 22:8 *"And Abraham said, My son, God will provide himself a lamb for a burnt offering: so they went both of them together."*

Ezekiel 46:13 *"Thou shalt daily prepare a burnt offering unto the Lord of a lamb of the first year without blemish: thou shalt prepare it every morning."*

John 1:29 *"The next day John seeth Jesus coming unto him, and saith, Behold the Lamb of God, which taketh away the sin of the world."*

"We learn to walk by stumbling." Bulgarian Proverb

EXPERIENCE,

    People can have their opinions and criticize my faith in You; however, no one can take away my very personal and private experiences with You during times where You have made Yourself very obvious and real to me. Thank You for all the times I have experienced You in special ways in my life. Also, I have found my experiences in life have been my greatest teachers of true wisdom and insight. I am not afraid to fall down every now and then because I know failures are only opportunities to learn and grow. You are more concerned with my character and growth than my comfort. Thank You for the good and the bad experiences that have taught me what I needed to learn to be a healthier me. I will intentionally follow Your course for my life.

    Love,
    Your Child

Ecclesiastes 1:16 *"I communed with mine own heart, saying, Lo, I am come to great estate, and have gotten more wisdom than all they that have been before me in Jerusalem: yea, my heart had great experience of wisdom and knowledge."*

"We all have weaknesses. But I have figured that others have put up with mine so tolerantly that I would be less than fair not to make a reasonable discount for theirs." William Allen White

NO RESPECTER OF PERSONS,

The ground is level at the foot of the cross. Everyone has a fair chance at salvation. No one is better than the other. No one is worse than the other. We all struggle with sin, and You hate all sin. You hate sin but love the sinner. I am an imperfect person who is in love with a Perfect God. I do not think I am so spiritual that I cannot fall. If I want people to forgive me when I fall then I need to show others the same respect. I need other people's help, and I should help everyone else in their journey. This teaches me to be fair and just in all of my relationships. I should not show favoritism. I should treat everyone fairly and equally, regardless of who they are, what their position is or what they have done in their past. I want everyone around me to feel valued, accepted and "a part of the group" in every setting I am in. Help me to treat everyone the same and not show favoritism.

Love,
Your Child

Acts 10:34 *"Then Peter opened his mouth, and said, Of a truth I perceive that God is no respecter of persons."*

> "Do not let what you cannot do interfere with what you can do." John Wooden

DIVINE INTERVENTION,

    Thank You for intervening in my life when I did not deserve Your help or was having a bad attitude. I pray Your love, mercy and grace would divinely intervene in the hopeless situations of those who are stuck in any sin or addiction. I pray for all those that need to let go of unhealthy, toxic people in their paths and do not know how to live without them. I pray You would divinely intervene and be who they need You to be. Please put new people in their path who are healthy for them, and please do the same in my life.

Love,
Your Child

Psalms 73:26 *"My flesh and my heart faileth: but God is the strength of my heart, and my portion for ever."*

Proverbs 13:20 *"He that walketh with wise men shall be wise: but a companion of fools shall be destroyed."*

> "There is a great difference between knowing a thing and understanding it."
> Charles Kettering with T.A. Boyd

CLARITY,

Please give me clear understanding of Your will and purpose in my life. Where there is confusion, let there be clarity. I pray for moments of clarity in other's lives when they are in the midst of chaos and confusion in their journey. When doctors, counselors or loved ones that You have placed in my life are talking to me, let me be open minded to the knowledge and insight that I need to make the necessary changes concerning my well-being. I know if I stay connected to You that I will receive a clear vision of Your will.

Love,
Your Child

1 Kings 3:10-12 "And the speech pleased the Lord, that Solomon had asked this thing. And God said unto him, Because thou hast asked this thing, and hast not asked for thyself long life: neither hast thou asked riches for thyself, nor hast thou asked the life of thine enemies; but hast asked for thyself understanding to discern judgment; Behold, I have done according to thy words: lo, I have given thee a wise and an understanding heart; so that there was none like thee before thee, neither after thee shall any arise like unto thee."

"Do not free a camel of the burden of his hump; you may be freeing him from being a camel." G.K. Chesterton

NECESSARY ONE,

You know what is necessary in my life. Some of the things I consider to be a burden are actually a blessing in disguise and are needed to lead me into my destiny. You also know what is unnecessary in my life. Because unnecessary things can bring about unnecessary pain, help me to rid myself of the unnecessary things that are keeping me from being a physically and emotionally healthy individual. I am responsible for my own health. It is not another's responsibility to ensure I am taking care of myself. If I need to make changes in my diet, give me the willingness and motivation to do so. If I need to start exercising, let me take the initiative. Show me what stressors are in my life that are hindering my health so I can walk away from them. It is Your will that I stay as healthy as I can. Let me love myself enough to see I am worth making any necessary changes to be healthy.

Love,
Your Child

Titus 3:14 *"And let ours also learn to maintain good works for necessary uses, that they be not unfruitful."*

> "One man practicing sportsmanship is far better than 50 preaching it."
> Knute K. Rockne

PREACHER,

You are my greatest preacher because You practiced what You taught. Help me to mirror Your example. I need to always have a preacher in my life to listen to. When I listen to a preacher teach and explain Your Word, it builds my faith. I will always need my faith built while living in this dark world. Keep Your hand on my preacher and his family.

Love,
Your Child

Romans 10:37 *"For whosoever shall call upon the name of the Lord shall be saved. How then shall they call on him in whom they have not believed? and how shall they believe in him of whom they have not heard? and how shall they hear without a preacher? And how shall they preach, except they be sent? as it is written, How beautiful are the feet of them that preach the gospel of peace, and bring glad tidings of good things! But they have not all obeyed the gospel. For Esaias saith, Lord, who hath believed our report? So then faith cometh by hearing, and hearing by the word of God.*

"Patience is bitter, but its fruit is sweet." Jean Jacques Rousseau

PATIENCE,

    I have peace and joy even in spite of the problems and sufferings of this life, if I know the trials, valleys, and tests I go through produce patience and perseverance in me with time. True joy comes from You, not circumstances, not material gain, not position and not power. I have joy in my journey because I have the Holy Ghost, which is Your Spirit living inside of me and enabling me to do what I need to do each day. This joy and contentment helps me to live patiently. Being impulsive is unhealthy and shows my impatience. Learning patience helps me to appreciate the things I have worked hard for and the things I have to wait for. You are so patient with me in my journey; let me also be patient with other people's journeys. You are working in all of our lives differently and we are all in different places in You. I will focus on the good in people and not focus on looking for what is wrong with people. What I struggle with may be someone else's strength and where they struggle may be my strength. I will love and respect people with where they are in their journey. I will not view people the way I met them but I will look at them according to how much they have grown since I met them.

Love,
Your Child

Roman 5:3 *"And not only so, but we glory in tribulations also: knowing that tribulation worketh patience . . ."*

Romans 14:17 *"For the kingdom of God is not meat and drink; but righteousness, and peace, and joy in the Holy Ghost."*

"Nothing so needs reforming as other people's habits." Mark Twain

HEALTHY ONE,

I know You want me to be healthy and whole in my mind, body and spirit. I pray to be free of sickness and disease, but I choose to trust You when my healing does not come while I am on earth. I pray for a sound mind and balance in my life. Please reveal to me anything I need to know that I may be doing that is hindering me from being healthy and whole. Help me to not ignore signs of illness that can be deadly if gone undetected. Give me the courage to overcome my fear and take the necessary tests to evaluate my health. Enable me to find the laughter each day offers because laughter boosts my immune system. I will drink water every day. I will go for a walk if I am able. I will make sure I am eating healthy. I will make sure I am getting at least eight hours of sleep a night. I will not eat too many sweets. I ask You bless all medicine I take and give my body favor with it. Let the medicines do what You want them to do in my body, without negative side effects. I will maintain healthy relationships and eliminate the stressors of unhealthy relationships from my life. I will do my part with what I can and trust that You will do Your part.

Love, Your Child

Exodus 20:12 "Honour thy father and thy mother: that thy days may be long upon the land which the Lord thy God giveth thee."

Proverbs 17:22 "A merry heart doeth good like a medicine: but a broken spirit drieth the bones."

Matthew 9:12 "But when Jesus heard that, he said unto them, They that be whole need not a physician, but they that are sick."

Day 52

"The most beautiful thing we can experience is the mysterious. It is the source of all true art and science." Albert Einstein

NEW TESTAMENT,

The new covenant of salvation, by which we are saved, is through Your death, burial and resurrection. We no longer have to sacrifice the blood of an animal to cover our sins until the "Messiah" comes, like they did in the Old Testament. Your blood, Lord Jesus, was shed when You became the perfect sacrifice of love. Therefore, the New Testament gives us the new plan of salvation because of You! Thank You for the opportunity to be saved!

Love,
Your Child

Hebrews 9:15 *"And for this cause he is the mediator of the new testament, that by means of death, for the redemption of the transgressions that were under the first testament, they which are called might receive the promise of eternal inheritance."*

> "Children are the living messages we send to a time we will not see."
> John W. Whitehead

NURTURER,

Help me to teach my children that You and Your ways should be a priority in their lives. Help me be a provider of food, clothing, education, protection and shelter. Let me teach them to be strong, independent adults with whom it is easy to get along with and be around. Let me be their biggest supporter to succeed in whatever You put in their hearts to do. Help me to allow them the freedom to make their own choices when they become adults instead of trying to control their decisions in order to get them to fulfill my will instead of Yours for their lives. Let me be an example to them while teaching them to live an abundant life. Let me teach them job skills and how to live within their means. Let me refrain from any type of abuse that could stunt my children's growth. Let me teach them to think outside the box, respect others, and to be givers, not takers. Let me teach them to not bully or make fun of others. Let me teach them how to tolerate being around many different types of people. If there is any area of my life where I felt neglected as a child, give me the ability to forgive my family and not use it as a crutch or excuse to not be the adult and example to my children that I am supposed to be. Let me nurture myself in those areas and receive Your healing.

Love,
Your Child

Psalms 27:10 *"When my father and my mother forsake me, then the Lord will take me up."*

Isaiah 49:15 *"Can a woman forget her sucking child, that she should not have compassion on the son of her womb? Yea, they may forget, yet will I not forget thee."*

"Blessed is the person who is too busy to worry in the daytime and too sleepy to worry at night." Leo Aikman

REFUGE,

You protect me from danger. When I am afraid, I will call on Your name. The acronym for fear is "False Evidence Appearing Real." It is the opposite of faith. You ease my worries and my fears. Worrying does nothing but waste my time and cause my heart to beat abnormally fast. I will put my worries and fears in Your hands, trusting You to do what only You can do. Instead of worrying, I will pray and live my life helping others, rather than drive myself crazy with something about which I can do nothing. Help me to focus on what I can do instead of what I have no control over.

Love,
Your Child

Psalms 46:1 *"God is our refuge and strength, a very present help in trouble."*

Psalms 91:1-5 *"He that dwelleth in the secret place of the most High shall abide under the shadow of the Almighty. I will say of the Lord, He is my refuge and my fortress: my God; in him will I trust. Surely he shall deliver thee from the snare of the fowler, and from the noisome pestilence. He shall cover thee with his feathers, and under his wings shalt thou trust: his truth shall be thy shield and buckler. Thou shalt not be afraid for the terror by night; nor for the arrow that flieth by day;"*

Psalms 91:10-11 *"There shall no evil befall thee, neither shall any plague come nigh thy dwelling. For he shall give his angels charge over thee, to keep thee in all thy ways."*

> "Don't tell me how hard you work. Tell me how much you get done."
> — James Ling

DEDICATED ONE,

I am dedicated to You and Your cause. In order for work to get done at its best, I have to be dedicated to the effort necessary to create the best outcome. Help me to do everything to the best of my ability, not halfheartedly. At school, let me study and be the best I can be. At my job, let me be indispensable and valuable to the company by going above and beyond in getting the work done, not just the minimum to get by. At church, let me focus on not just getting what I need from You, but praying and supporting others with their needs. I want to be reliable, dependable and loyal to those around me. My words and actions impact all those around me so I want my actions to reflect Your character and will. Let me do everything You put in front of me with a good attitude.

Love,
Your Child

Ecclesiastes 9:10 *"What so ever thy hand findeth to do, do with thy might; for there is no work, nor device, nor knowledge, nor wisdom in the grave, whether thou goest."*

2 Chronicles 5:1 *"Thus all the work that Solomon made for the house of the Lord was finished: and Solomon brought in all the things that David his father had dedicated; and the silver, and the gold, and the instruments, put he among the treasures of the house of God."*

"Our prayers are answered not when we are given what we ask but when we are challenged to be what we can be." Morris Adler

DOER,

You are the way, the truth and the life. When I pray in secret, unplugged from the world around me, that is where I draw my inner strength from You. We have a special, intimate relationship. It is the battles I fight privately in prayer where I obtain what is needed when I am in public. There are some things that do not need to be shared with anyone but You. You share Your insight and secrets with me when I am alone with You. You show me what direction to take. At the same time, I pray You will shut doors and open doors in accordance to Your will and timing. Give me the restraint to not open a door that You want closed and the discernment to not slam a door shut that You are trying to open. I choose to be a "doer," not just a "hearer." Help me to both do and accept Your will.

Love,
Your Child

Matthew 6:6 *"But thou, when thou prayest, enter into the closet, and when thou hast shut thy door, pray to thy Father which is in secret; and thy Father which seeth in secret shall reward thee openly."*

James 1:22 *"But be ye doers of the word, and not hearers only, deceiving your own selves."*

"Conscience is God's presence in man." **Emanuel Swedenborg**

GOSPEL,

There are four gospels: Matthew, Mark, Luke and John. They each give an account of Your life on this earth. If we were to have four people, each with a different background, go outside at the same time and describe the blue sky, they would all describe it in their own way; however, their opinions would not change the fact the sky is blue. It is the same way with the four gospels. The message is the same but described differently. Help me to spread Your message of love in the special way only I can. Some are gifted in song, some are able to spread Your message in teaching, and others can render medical aid. Some are missionaries, some are counselors, and some minister in prisons. We all come from different backgrounds and are able to show Your love in so many different ways. Help me to be sensitive to Your voice and leading while living out Your message. Let my example of doing what is right be what people see, not just what I have to say. The message of the cross, Your parables and teachings are what I want to practice.

Love, Your Child

Luke 4:18 *"The Spirit of the Lord is upon me, because he hath anointed me to preach the gospel to the poor; he hath sent me to heal the brokenhearted, to preach deliverance to the captives, and receiving of sight to the blind, to set at liberty they that are bruised."*

1 Corinthians 12:12 *"For as the body is one, and hath many members, and all the members of that one body, being many, are one body: so also is Christ."*

2 Corinthians 3:2 *"Ye are our epistle written in our hearts, known and read of all men."*

> "Gossip needn't be false to be evil—there's a lot of truth that shouldn't be passed around." Frank A. Clark

BLESSING,

You are my greatest blessing, and You are enough. I want to be a blessing to others! Quicken my spirit before I open my mouth and say something I may regret. I do not want to participate in gossip just to feel like part of the group. I do not want to gossip out of jealousy in order to feel superior to someone else by tearing down the good that they are trying to accomplish. I do not want to gossip out of boredom either. I also do not want to curse people by gossiping or speaking negatively about them. It is character assassination. Help me not to put people down or belittle them. I want to focus on the best in people and protect their reputations. I want to speak blessings over people's lives and be an encourager when they fall. Let me be a blessing, not a curse, to You, others and myself.

Love, Your Child

Numbers 6:22-27 "And the Lord spake unto Moses, saying, Speak unto Aaron and unto his sons, saying, On this wise ye shall bless the children of Israel, saying unto them, The Lord bless thee, and keep thee: The Lord make his face shine upon thee, and be gracious unto thee: The Lord light up his countenance upon thee, and give thee peace. And they shall put my name upon the children of Israel; and I will bless them."

James 3:9-11 "Therewith bless we God, even the Father; and therewith curse we men; which are made after the similitude of God. Out of the same mouth proceedeth blessing and cursing. My brethren, these things ought not so to be. Doth a fountain send forth at the same place sweet water and bitter?"

> "To have a right to do a thing is not at all the same as to be right in doing it."
> G.K. Chesterton

GATE,

I will open my day with a spirit of gratitude, reminding myself to live in Your righteous ways. Remind me as I face the day that I am the one who is in charge of how I allow people to talk to me or treat me. My reactions to people define what are acceptable and unacceptable behaviors. It is okay to say "yes," but it is also okay to say "no," without explanation. Setting limits is healthy. I know that the boundaries necessary for my emotional and physical health may be unnecessary for someone else. Boundaries are for protection. Boundaries keep order in my life. It is my responsibility to build and maintain the boundaries I need to have. I cannot allow some things or people into my life because it is unhealthy for my well-being. Help me to respect other people's boundaries as I would want them to respect mine.

Love,
Your Child

Psalms 118:19-21 *"Open to me the gates of righteousness: I will go into them, and I will praise the Lord: This gate of the Lord, into which the righteous shall enter. I will praise thee: for thou hast heard me, and art become my salvation."*

> "Waiting is still an occupation. It is not having anything to wait for that is terrible." Cesare Pavese

WATCHER,

Thank You for looking out for me. Today, I choose to pay attention to whatever You want to say to me or through me to someone else. I am guarding my heart from accepting sin. I am staying away from my personal triggers that could lead me to be tempted to do wrong. I will not react to my emotional triggers. I will not allow my triggers to lead me back to a place in my life that I do not need to revisit. I am watching for anything trying to block me from moving forward, all the while watching for You.

Love,
Your Child

Matthew 26:40-41 *"And he cometh unto the disciples, and findeth them asleep, and saith unto Peter, What, could ye not watch with me one hour? Watch and pray, that ye enter not into temptation: the spirit indeed is willing, but the flesh is weak."*

"Get down on your knees and thank God you are on your feet." Irish saying

NOTHING IS TOO HARD,

I will not lose sight of the reality that nothing is too hard for You. You can change my situation at any time You feel like it. I know You know what is best for me. I will stay focused on the fact that Your plan is the bigger picture. I will trust in Your plan and submit to it, whether I agree or disagree. You are the Lord of my life, not me. I love You.

Love,
Your Child

Jeremiah 32:17 "Ah Lord God! behold, thou hast made the heaven and the earth by thy great power and stretched and arm, and there is nothing too hard for thee:"

Matthew 19:26 "But Jesus beheld them, and said unto them, With men this is impossible; but with God all things are possible."

"He that would be a leader must be a bridge." Welsh Proverb

LEADERSHIP,

You made a way out of no way for me. When I burnt bridges with people when I was not healthy, You made a way for reconciliation. When I purposely shut You out of my life, You made a way back into my life. When diagnosed with an illness, You made a way through medication. When I was headed to a dark place, Your light made a way for my deliverance. When I chose to get baptized in Your Name, Jesus, it was my way of saying that I not only want forgiveness, I also want You to lead my life because my will messes everything up. What You did on the Cross built the bridge for me to be able to get to You. I will acknowledge You in all of my decisions and follow Your ways. As You lead me, I will lead others to You.

Love,
Your Child

Proverbs 3:6 *"In all thy ways acknowledge him, and he shall direct thy paths."*

"Progress begins with the belief that what is necessary is possible."
— **Norman Cousins**

JEHOVAH JIREH,

You are my provider. You know my needs. If something is taken away from me that I need, I know You will provide something in its place at the right time. You use many different avenues to provide, and You are always right on time. Thank You for being my constant provider with the unlimited resources of Heaven.

Love,
Your Child

Genesis 22:13-14 *"And Abraham lifted up his eyes, and looked, and behold behind him a ram caught in a thicket by his horns: and Abraham went and took the ram, and offered him up for a burnt offering in the stead of his son. And Abraham called the name of that place Jehovahjireh: as it is said to this day, In the mount of the Lord it shall be seen."*

"Nothing lasts forever—not even your troubles." Arnold H. Glasow

WONDERFUL,

I love everything about You! You truly are wonderful. I know life has its ups and downs. Life is full of mountain top experiences and valleys. Some days are good, and some days are bad. This makes life such a wonderful challenging adventure! I am not afraid of the challenges of life. The bad days are what make the good days so wonderful. If every day was a good day, I would probably take You for granted and I would not look forward to going to Heaven. On my bad days, I will remind myself of the times of deliverance, healing, protection and victory of the good days. I also know that not every day is a bad day. I know that feelings come and go according to our circumstances. When I feel bad, that feeling will eventually pass.

Love,
Your Child

Psalms 119:129 *"Thy testimonies are wonderful: therefore doth my soul keep them."*

"Most people want to be delivered from temptation but would like it to keep in touch." Robert Orben

MAINTENANCE,

You have the power to deliver me from addictions and sins of all kinds; however, temptation will always come in many forms to try to take me off my path. Therefore, it is my responsibility to maintain my deliverance and recovery by being proactive in taking the steps necessary to continue my journey of wholeness.

Love,
Your Child

Titus 3:7-8 *"That being justified by his grace, we should be made heirs according to the hope of eternal life. This is a faithful saying, and these things I will that they affirm constantly, that they which have believed in God might be careful to maintain good works. These things are good and profitable unto men."*

> "Liberty, when it begins to take root, is a plant of rapid growth."
> — George Washington

THE ONE WHO REIGNS,

I want Your Spirit to control and reign over every area of my life. I do not want to be controlled by a toxic relationship, food, drugs, alcohol, cigarettes, anxiety, fear, depression, or obsessive thoughts. I only want to be led by You. I do not want sin to control me. Lord, rule and reign over every part of my heart, life, thoughts, motives, words and actions today.

Love,
Your Child

Romans 6:11-13 *"Likewise reckon ye also yourselves to be dead indeed unto sin, but alive unto God through Jesus Christ our Lord. Let not sin therefore reign in your mortal body, that ye should obey it in the lusts thereof. Neither yield ye your members as instruments of unrighteousness unto sin: but yield yourselves unto God, as those that are alive from the dead, and your members as instruments of righteousness unto God."*

"It's a funny thing about life; if you refuse to accept anything but the best, you very often get it." W. Somerset Maugham

BAPTIZER,

I am glad I am a believer who is baptized in Your Name. Creator, Father, Son, Savior and Holy Ghost are common nouns and titles. JESUS is Your Name. It is a proper noun. I know when I made the decision to be baptized in the name of the One who died for my sins that it not only means my sins are forgiven, but that I choose to live for You. You, Jesus, are the one to whom I am meant to submit my life. I want to stay away from my old, sinful nature which died at my baptism. Now with Your resurrection power, I can begin living in Your nature and character.

Love, Your Child

Deuteronomy 6:4 "Hear, O Israel: The Lord our God is one Lord."

Matthew 28:19 "Go ye therefore, and teach all nations, baptizing them in the name of the Father, and of the Son, and of the Holy Ghost."

Mark 16:16 "He that believeth and is baptized shall be saved; but he that believeth not shall be damned."

Luke 3:16 "John answered, saying unto them all, I indeed baptize you with water, but one mightier than I cometh, the latchet of whose shoes I am not worthy to unloose: he shall baptize you with the Holy Ghost and with fire."

John 10:30 "I and my Father are one."

Acts 2:38 "Then Peter said unto them, Repent, and be baptized every one of you in the name of Jesus Christ for the remission of sins, and ye shall receive the gift of the Holy Ghost."

Ephesians 4:5 "One Lord, one faith, one baptism."

"**The three hardest tasks in the world are neither physical feats nor intellectual achievements, but moral acts: to return love for hate, to include the excluded, and to say, 'I was wrong.'"** Sydney J. Harris

BANNER,

    Your Banner over me is love. You included me when I excluded You. You included me when I was excluded by others. There are many unfair reasons why people exclude others. I know what it feels like to be "left out," whether it is because of my past failures, or because I do not dress a certain way, or because I am not in a certain social class. I know the feeling of rejection and hurt. I remember how much I wanted to feel "a part of" the group. Because I know this feeling too well, I do not want anyone around me to feel this way in my presence. Therefore, I will go out of my way to make sure everyone around me feels valued. Forgive me for any time I may have excluded one of Your children in any setting. You can love through me in such a way that people will be drawn to You because You are love. Your Word boldly proclaims Your love for me. Your love is permanent and unconditional. It never changes or waivers because of my circumstances or actions. Your love will never leave me no matter what I say or do. I belong to You. I can be secure in Your love for me. Forgive me for the times I have doubted Your love.

Love,
Your Child

Song of Solomon 2:4 *"He brought me to the banqueting house, and his banner over me was love."*

1 John 4:7-8 *"Beloved, let us love one another: for love is of God; and every one that loveth is born of God; and knoweth God. He that loveth not knoweth not God; for God is love."*

> "When there is an original sound in the world, it wakens a hundred echoes."
> John A. Shedd

NAZARITE,

You are Holy. The Nazarites in the Old Testament lived a very separated lifestyle that stood out to everyone. For instance, they did not drink wine, they did not cut their hair, and they were to have no contact with dead bodies or graves. I know as a Christian that my words, dress, behaviors and reactions should be different from those who do not know You. You want me to be separate and different from others. You want my conversations to be honest, uplifting, and Godly. You want me to protect my spirit from things that can pollute it. Help me to be separate and Holy. I am consecrated to You. Help me to stand out for You. Give me the courage to go against the grain of society when it comes to doing the right thing.

Love,
Your Child

Numbers 6:2-8 "Speak unto the children of Israel, and say unto them, When either man or woman shall separate themselves to vow a vow of a Nazarite, to separate themselves unto the Lord: He shall separate himself from wine and strong drink, and shall drink no vinegar of wine, or vinegar of strong drink, neither shall he drink any liquor of grapes, nor eat moist grapes, or dried. All the days of his separation shall he eat nothing that is made of the vine tree, from the kernels even to the husk. All the days of the vow of his separation there shall no razor come upon his head: until the days be fulfilled, in that which he separateth himself unto the Lord, he shall be holy, and shall let the locks of the hair of his head grow. All the days that he seperateth himself unto the Lord he shall come at no dead body. He shall not make himself unclean for his father, or for his mother, for his brother, or for his sister, when they die: because the consecration of his God is upon his head. All the days of his separation he is holy unto the Lord."

1 Peter 1:14-16 "As obedient children, not fashioning yourselves according to the former lusts in your ignorance: But as he which hath called you is holy, so be ye holy in all manner of conversation; because it is written, Be ye holy; for I am holy."

> "People who drink to drown their sorrow should be told that sorrow knows how to swim." Ann Landers

ACQUAINTED WITH GRIEF,

Thank You that there is no emotion You have not felt. You can relate to our deepest sorrows. When my heart is heavy and there are hot tears streaming uncontrollably down my face, You are with me and can relate. When it came time for You to bear my Cross, enduring great emotional and physical suffering, You experienced every feeling I have felt, but at a horrible extreme I cannot imagine. You were rejected by someone very close to You who was embarrassed and afraid to be connected to You during Your darkest time. You were made fun of, laughed at and spat on. You were misunderstood by the political leaders of that day. You were physically tortured in the worst way. You were humiliated in front of everyone by being nailed naked to the Cross. I am glad You did not allow Your circumstances to stop You from fulfilling the "Big Picture." Because of Your perfect yet costly sacrifice, I have a chance at both redemption and eternity. You are acquainted with grief. Everyone feels the same emotions in life; it is just different circumstances that bring out those emotions. I know when I am feeling bad or low I have to continue moving forward in my life no matter what. I cannot be controlled by my emotions. I have to be led by what I know to do. I have to stay active and live my life, even when everything in me wants to isolate and hide in bed. I cannot allow my grief to turn into a pity party. I need to have a good cry and then choose to move on. And I will. I know feelings come and go and I will not feel the way I presently feel forever.

Love, Your Child

Isaiah 53:3-4 *"He is despised and rejected of men; a man of sorrows, and acquainted with grief: and we hid as it were our faces from him; he was despised, and we esteemed him not. Surely he hath borne our griefs, and carried our sorrows: yet we did esteem him stricken, smitten of God, and afflicted."*

> "Happiness, I have discovered, is nearly always a rebound from hard work."
> David Grayson

GIVER OF PURPOSE,

Please reveal to me Your purpose for my life. I do know that You are a lover of all people. Loving people is the ultimate part of Your purpose, and, therefore, my purpose too. I also know that whatever You put in front of me each day to do, I should do it to the best of my ability. I will listen to that still, small voice inside of me leading me on my way. Help me to adjust quickly when life throws me a curve ball. Help me to not be bitter and frustrated at Your divine detours and interruptions during my journey, whether it be sickness, a job change, a loss, or a simple divine delay. I will fulfill whatever my purpose is the best I can. If it is mentoring people in recovery from addictions, let me be sincerely involved in their lives. If it is being a nurse, let me care for the patients the way I would want to be cared for. If it is being a mechanic, let me do a thorough job so people will be safe in their vehicles. If it is to be a school bus driver, let me put a smile on each child's face who I come across. If it is to be an intercessory prayer warrior, praying for Your will, protection and healing in other people's lives, let me be passionate about it.

Love, Your Child

Ecclesiastes 3:1 *"To every thing there is a season, and a time to every purpose under the Heaven."*

Ecclesiastes 9:10 *"Whatsoever thy hand findeth to do, do it with thy might; for there is no work, nor device, nor knowledge, nor wisdom in the grave, whither thou goest."*

"Say what you have to say, not what you ought." Henry David Thoreau

ARK OF THE COVENANT,

You always make me think of the secret, intimate places in prayer behind the veil. It is a private place where I can safely share my secrets. In the Tabernacle Plan of the Old Testament the Ark of the Covenant was behind the veil, where only the High Priest could go. The ark was a box made of acacia wood and covered in gold. Aaron's rod that budded and the Ten Commandments, or the law, was placed inside the Ark of the Covenant. It was covered by the mercy seat, with an angel on each side of the mercy seat. The location of the mercy seat represented Your mercy covering the law. The blood of the sacrificed animal was sprinkled by the High Priest onto the mercy seat. It is where You revealed Yourself to the High Priest and where You revealed Your secrets. Before You went to the Cross, Your children only had access to You through the High Priest. You tore the veil in the temple in the New Testament through Your perfect sinless sacrifice on the Cross. The torn veil symbolizes we now have direct access to You and no longer have to hear from You through the High Priest. I long to go to the secret place in prayer where I am changed by Your Presence and share my secrets while hoping You will share Your secrets with me.

Love, Your Child

1 Samuel 4:5 *"And when the ark of the covenant of the Lord came into the camp, all Isreal shouted with a great shout, so that the earth rang again."*

1 Chronicles 22:19 *"Now set your heart and your soul to seek the Lord your God; arise therefore, and build ye the sanctuary of the Lord God, to bring the ark of the covenant of the Lord, and the holy vessels of God, into the House that is to be built to the name of the Lord."*

Mark 15:38 *"And the veil of the temple was rent in twain from the top to the bottom."*

"Our language has wisely sensed the two sides of being alone. It has created the word 'loneliness' to express the pain of being alone. And it has created the word 'solitude' to express the glory of being alone." Paul Tillich

EMMANUEL,

When I feel lonely, help me to remember the reality of Your Word that says You are always with me. I can pray, listen to worship music and enjoy Your presence. I can take the alone time that is given to me to also nurture and take care of myself. You are with me as I go through the ups and downs of this life. I need You and do not want to try to go through this life without You.

Love,
Your Child

Mathew 1:23 *"Behold, a virgin shall be with child, and shall bring forth a son, and they shall call his name Emmanuel, which being interpreted is, God with us."*

Day 74

> "If you would thoroughly know anything, teach it to others." Tyron Edwards

EDIFYER,

I know You want me to grow up and mature in ALL areas of my life. I also know that we as Christians should edify each other. We should do it with a heart of love, not be mean-spirited. We all need each other. Let my relationships with others be healthy and point me to You and Your ways. We should not draw people away from You but draw people toward You and what is right. We need You to be able to do the next right thing because what is right is not always the first thing that comes to mind.

Love,
Your Child

Ephesians 4:12 *"For the perfecting of the saints, for the work of the ministry, for the edifying of the body of Christ."*

Ephesians 4:16 *"From whom the whole body fitly joined together and compacted by that which every joint supplieth, according to the effectual working in the measure of every part, maketh increase of the body unto the edifying of itself in love."*

> "Of course, it's the same old story. Truth usually is the same old story."
> — Margaret Thatcher

TESTIMONY,

Your message stays the same. Because of Your testimony, I have an overcoming testimony. Therefore, when I am facing challenging circumstances I will always remind myself of the past victories that You have won in my life. I will also share an encouraging word with others of all the wonderful things that You have done in my life. You encourage me, so I should encourage others. I overcome and keep the victory by Your blood and by sharing with others my story of Your grace which is very alive in my life.

Love,
Your Child

Revelation 12:11 *"And they overcame him by the blood of the Lamb, and by the word of their testimony; and they loved not their lives unto the death."*

"He who sings frightens away his ills." Miguel DeCervantes Saevedra

My Song,

One of the ways I pray is by listening to Your music and singing songs of praise to You. Music can be very healthy for me. It lowers anxiety and stress and motivates me when I am exercising. It increases the blood flow in my blood vessels. When my mind is not in a good place, I can change my mood by listening to wholesome, uplifting music about You. I can sing to You. I know You love it when I sing to You and You do not care what I sound like because You love that it is coming from my heart.

Love,
Your Child

Psalm 28:7 *"The Lord is my strength and my shield; my heart trusted in him, and I am helped: therefore my heart greatly rejoiceth; and with my song will I praise him."*

"There is no surprise more magical than the surprise of being loved. It is God's finger on man's shoulder." Charles Morgan

SPONTANEOUS,

You continually show up in my life in so many ways. I love it when You spontaneously surprise me with an unexpected answered prayer or with Your sweet presence meeting me where I am. It is as if You are blowing kisses to me from heaven. Thank You for all the sweet things that You do to remind me that You are alive in my life! I do not want to believe in my perceived reality. I want to believe in Your spontaneous reality. So let Your reality become my reality.

Love,
Your Child

Jeremiah 51:41 *"How is Sheshach taken! and how is the praise of the whole earth surprised! how is Babylon become an astonishment among the nations!"*

"There is nothing stronger in the world than gentleness." Hans Suyin

GENTLE,

Just because I am in pain or having a bad day does not give me the right to take my frustration out on those around me. My sickness is my battle to fight, not theirs. Help me to be aware of how I come across to others and take responsibility for my own emotions and behaviors. I do not want to be forceful, arrogant, rough or harsh in my demeanor or tone of voice because of my own personal frustrations. I want to be able to understand where other people are coming from. I want to be approachable. Help me to have Your gentle ways.

Love,
Your Child

1 Thessalonians 2:7 *"But we were gentle among you, even as a nurse cherisheth her children."*

Galatians 5:22-25 *"But the fruit of the Spirit is love, joy, peace, longsuffering, gentleness, goodness, faith, meekness, temperance: against such there is no law. And they that are Christ's have crucified the flesh with the affections and lusts. If we live in the Spirit, let us also walk in the Spirit."*

> "The way I see it, if you want the rainbow, you gotta put up with the rain."
> **Dolly Parton**

RAIN,

    Help me to understand and accept that bad things happen to everyone sometimes. You say it rains on the just and the unjust. It is a part of life. It is all about how I respond to the storm and my attitude while enduring life's winds and rains. Eventually, the storm will pass; it will not last forever. The sun will always come out again.

    Love,
    Your Child

Matthew 5:45 *"That ye may be the children of your Father which is in Heaven: for he maketh his sun to rise on the evil and on the good, and sendeth rain on the just and the unjust."*

"Extending your hand is extending yourself." Rod McKuen

FAVOR,

When I am in Your will I have favor with You. Everything falls into place and everyone that is needed to make Your dream for my life a reality comes together beautifully. Grant me favor to have victory over the enemy the way David had victory when defeating Goliath. Grant me the kind of protective favor that baby Moses had with the Pharaoh's daughter. Grant me the favor that Mary had to be the willing vessel through which You came into this world as a baby. Grant me the favor Joseph had in the end with his brothers after he was betrayed by them in his younger years. Grant me favor in my intercessory prayers for my loved ones the way Abraham had in his prayers for Lot. Grant me the favor of Your grace that Paul had with You to not allow the thorn in the flesh to hinder him from fulfilling Your will for his life. I pray favor with You and everyone I come across. I love You much.

Love,
Your Child

Job 1:12 "Thou has granted me life and favour, and thy visitation hath preserved my spirit."

2 Corinthians 12:7-10 "And lest I should be exalted above measure through the abundance of the revelations, there way given to me a thorn in the flesh, the messenger of Satan to buffet me, lest I should be exalted above measure. For this thing I besought the Lord thrice, that it might depart from me. And he said unto me, My grace is sufficient for thee: for my strength is made perfect in weakness. Most gladly therefore will I rather glory in my infirmities, that the power of Christ may rest upon me. Therefore I take pleasure in infirmities, in reproaches, in necessities, in persecutions, in distresses for Christ's sake: for when I am weak, then am I strong."

"The reward for work well done is the opportunity to do more." Jonas Salk

THE ONE WHO DOES GOOD WORKS,

    My actions speak way louder than my words or beliefs. Let my actions make a positive statement. Let my actions line up with my beliefs of You and Your Word. One of the ways I let my light shine is through my good works. Let me be mindful of how my actions affect those around me. I know that I am not saved by my good works, but because I love You, I want to please You by doing good works.

    Love,
    Your Child

Matthew 5:16 *"Let your light so shine before men, that they may see your good works, and glorify your Father which is in heaven."*

Ephesians 2:10 *"For we are his workmanship, created in Christ Jesus unto good works, which God hath before ordained that we should walk in them."*

"Growing up is usually so painful that people make comedies out of it to soften the memory." John Greenwald

HEART MENDER,

A broken heart can manifest itself as physical pain, leading to high blood pressure and an increased heart rate, which puts people at risk of a heart attack. This is why I need Your help to process my grief in a healthy manner. When my heart is broken into what seems like a million pieces, I know that You are safe and that I can trust You with my deepest pain. I can unleash my tears to You in prayer. When I'm grieving, put people or things in my path that will make me laugh. I will look for the jokes life has to offer when going through a trial and will help others see the funny parts of life too. When other people are hurting, let my words heal their hearts and let me be Your voice in helping them deal with their losses. I will not judge someone for how long it takes them to grieve a loss or how they choose to process their pain. I will check on them periodically to make sure they know I care. I will try to help them with whatever they need. Help me be someone else's healing. You heal me when I allow myself to be Your healing hands and feet.

Love,
Your Child

Psalm 147:3 *"He healeth the broken in heart, and bindeth up their wounds."*

Proverbs 17:22 *"A merry heart doeth good like a medicine: but a broken spirit drieth up the bones."*

Luke 4:18 *"The Spirit of the Lord is upon me, because he hath anointed me to preach the gospel to the poor, he hath sent me to heal the brokenhearted, to preach deliverance to the captives, and recovering of sight to the blind, to set at liberty them that are bruised."*

"What you have inherited from your fathers, earn over again for yourselves, or it will not be yours." Johann Wolfgang von Goethe

DAVID'S OFFSPRING,

You are not only the promised Messiah coming from the lineage of David, You are also the Creator of David and all things. You are able to fulfill many roles at the same time. Joseph came from the lineage of David, and Mary's father came from the lineage of David. Because I am baptized in You, I am Your child, which makes me royalty and part of David's offspring, which means I get to receive all of the wonderful promises that goes along with being in Your family.

Love,
Your Child

Deuteronomy 7:9 *"Know therefore that the Lord thy God, he is God, the faithful God, which keepeth covenant and mercy with them that love him and keep his commandments to a thousand generations."*

Matthew 1:1 *"The book of the generation of Jesus Christ, the son of David, the son of Abraham."*

Luke 3:32 *"Which was the son of Jesse, which was the son of Obed, which was the son of Booz, which is the son of Salmon, which was the son of Naasson."*

Revelation 22:16 *"I Jesus have sent mine angel to testify unto you these things in the churches. I am the root and the offspring of David, and the bright and morning star."*

"You don't get to choose how you're going to die. Or when. You can only decide how you're going to live now." Joan Baez

ETERNAL,

It is so good to know that life is not limited to what this earth has to offer. I will motivate myself the way David did when everything was coming against him, including his very own people. I will depend on Your guidance and not other people's opinions for my life because You see the beginning from the end. Your view is unlimited compared to our limited view of life. I will move forward as each day goes by, and will stay focused on the eternal purpose. I will do my best to bring value to my job, church and community because it all plays a part in Your eternal plan. I cannot wait to meet You face to face. The first thing I want to do, if possible, is give You a big hug! Until that day, I pray to know You more intimately as each day passes. I cannot wait to spend forever and ever with You, the lover of my soul!

Love, Your Child

1 Samuel 30:6 *"And David was greatly distressed; for the people spake of stoning him, because the soul of all the people was grieved, every man for his sons and for his daughters: but David encouraged himself in the Lord his God."*

John 3:16 *"That whosoever believeth in him should not perish, but have eternal life."*

John 17:3 *"And this is life eternal, that they might know thee the only true God, and Jesus Christ, whom thou hast sent."*

"The most important thing a father can do for his children is to love their mother." Theodore Hesburgh

HEAD OF THE CHURCH,

Your Spirit and voice should lead all ministry decisions because You are the Head of the Church. It is made up of members from all over this world. Every person plays a part in expanding Your kingdom. Every part is important and necessary. The same way You love Your church, so much that You gave Your life for it, is the same way husbands should love their wives. Remind us of this.

Love,
Your Child

Ephesians 5:23 *"For the husband is the head of the wife, even as Christ is the head of the church: and he is the savior of the body."*

Ephesians 5:25 *"Husbands, love your wives, even as Christ also loved the church, and gave himself for it."*

"Perseverance is the hard work you do after you get tired of doing the hard work you already did." Newt Gingrich

STRENGTH,

There are times I feel so drained that I do not know how I am supposed to make it through the day. When I call on Your name, I know You will divinely intervene and impart special supernatural strength for me to accomplish Your will. You equip those who You call. When I feel that extra special strength come out of nowhere, that is when I know You have stepped in and become who I need You to be to get through the day. Thank You for the assurance strength is on its way.

Love,
Your Child

Isaiah 40:29 *"He giveth power to the faint; and to them that have no might he increaseth strength."*

> "If you begin to live life looking for the God that is all around you, every moment becomes a prayer." Frank Bianco

PRESENCE,

I seek You. I know if I am looking for You I will find You. In Your presence, I am comforted and find peace. In Your presence, I am spiritually restored and strengthened. In Your presence, I hear Your voice and know I am not alone. In Your presence, I see that I matter and have value. In Your presence, I am forgiven and am granted an opportunity to try again. In Your presence, I receive spiritual surgery for my heart that transforms my motives and my perspective. In Your presence, I am being healed and made whole. But I have to look for You. I do not want to go anywhere without Your presence going before me. In Your presence, I truly find everything I need. If I have nothing but You, then I have everything because You are everything.

Love,
Your Child

Exodus 33:15 *"And he said unto him, if thy presence go not with me, carry us not up hence."*

"The intelligent man who is proud of his intelligence is like the condemned man who is proud of his large cell." Simone Weil

SUCCESS,

I know You want me to be successful and to live an abundant life. You want me to do everything to the best of my ability; however, You do not want me to become haughty when succeeding in life. I am only blessed with success because of You, not by my own power. You give me the ability to succeed. You can take away my abilities to perform at any time. I am not better than others for any reason. We all have different giftings that are equally important to getting the job done. We are all level at the foot of the Cross. We are all important and have value because You give us value.

Love,
Your Child

Proverbs 16:18 *"Pride goeth before destruction, and an haughty spirit before a fall."*

Ecclesiastes 9:10 *"Whatsoever thy hand findeth to do, do it with thy might; for there is no work, nor device, nor knowledge, nor wisdom in the grave, whither thou goest."*

"In quiet places, reason abounds." Adlai E. Stevenson

QUIETNESS,

To start my day off right, I have to spend quiet time alone with You first. I need to fill my mind up with You and Your thoughts so that I am so full of You that the evils of the day have no place to pollute my mind and spirit. I can start my day filling myself up with You and going over my schedule for the day. When busy, remind me that I need to get away from everything and embrace the quiet. I will shut out the noise. I do not have to be afraid to be alone with my own thoughts. I will not waste time rehearsing my failures during my quiet time with You. I will make sense of what is going on inside of me and around me. I will discern what to let go of and what to consider. I have to find time to quietly rejuvenate. A few moments to myself daily is necessary for good health. Therefore, I will be still, breathe and let You unfold Your Plan to me.

Love,
Your Child

Psalms 23:2 *"He maketh me to lie down in green pastures: he leadeth Me beside the still waters."*

Psalms 46:10 *"Be still, and know that I am God: I will be exalted among the heathen, I will be exalted in the earth."*

"The only way to keep your health is to eat what you don't want, drink what you don't like, and do what you druther not." Mark Twain

PRIORITY,

Keeping You first is a goal I must set daily because I struggle being consistently balanced. How I spend my time is valuable; I do not want my time wasted. I know my well-being has to be a top priority. I will make a weekly goal list of what I know is most important in my life and make time in my schedule to fulfill those necessary goals. I will get rid of any toxic relationships that provide only negative influences that distract my time from Your purpose. I will pay my bills on time, while saving for emergencies. I will manage my time well with household chores so that things do not get out of hand. I will make the proper adjustments necessary to adapt to any medication I have to take so that it can do what it is supposed to do inside my body. I will take a time of refreshing for myself so I can be who You need me to be when I am around Your children. Help me to keep my priorities straight and to keep You first.

Love,
Your Child

Matthew 6:33 *"But seek ye first the Kingdom of God, and his righteousness; and all these things shall be added unto you."*

> "Let freedom reign. The sun never set on so glorious a human achievement."
> -Nelson Mandela

Sun,

Every day I wake up is a gift from You. In the spiritual, You are my source of light that brightens my path for the day. You shine on the areas of my life to show me where I need to be free of anyone or anything stopping me from being who I need to be. To be free is to be spiritually whole. In the natural, I need to have sunlight sometimes to absorb Vitamin D for my health. The sunlight can even help my mood. So, I will open all of the windows in my life, the natural windows to let the sunlight in and the windows of my heart to allow You to come in and shine to bring healing, freedom, and light to guide me.

Love,
Your Child

Psalms 84:11 *"For the Lord God is a sun and shield: the Lord will give grace and glory: no good thing will he withhold from them that walk upright."*

"Normal day, let me be aware of the treasure you are." Mary Jean Irion

TREASURE,

It is a shame we can spend our lives daily looking for something or someone that can give us satisfaction, when the answer is with us every day. You are the answer. You are my ultimate treasure. When I seek You and listen to what You are speaking to my heart, I find the treasures You want me to find. Each day I am with "The Treasure"—You—who gives me the gift of the present moment to enjoy. I will not waste the gift of another day You have given me by allowing it to be unproductive. I will not waste my precious treasure of a day by having a bad attitude or feeling sorry for myself for the condition I am presently living with. My greatest decision is the attitude I choose to have for each day. Each health condition can uncover a treasure in my life I did not realize was there if it were not for the challenge I am facing. Sometimes the treasure is hidden or disguised as a trial that uncovers and unfolds itself as an unexpected gift that is truly a treasure. I will choose to look for the treasure in the trial.

Love,
Your Child

Mathew 6:21 *"For where your treasure is, there will your heart be also."*

Mathew 13:44 *"Again, the kingdom of heaven is like unto treasure hidden in a field; that which when a man hath found, he hideth, and for joy thereof goeth and selleth all that he hath, and buyeth that field."*

> "Excuses are the nails used to build a house of failure."
> — Don Wilder and Bill Rechin

My HEALTH,

It is Your will that I be as healthy as I can be. I need to take the best care of my body which houses Your Spirit. I have a "no excuses" attitude. Excuses are only a justification for me to feel better about doing something I know I have no business doing. There is no excuse to hurt someone else, not take care of the condition I am in, or to willingly do wrong. If I do participate in something I need to apologize to someone about, I will own my part in it and not give excuses for my poor behavior. I love myself and my future so much I am not willing to put anything into my body that has the potential to destroy my destiny. I refuse to allow myself to become stressed out by allowing toxic and negative people to influence me. I will do whatever it takes, with Your Power that works in me to take responsibility for my choices and my attitude.

Love,
Your Child

1 Corinthians 6:19-20 *"What? Know ye not that your body is the temple of the Holy Ghost which is in you, which ye have of God, and ye are not your own? For ye are bought with a price; therefore glorify God in your body, and in your spirit, which are God's."*

"**Resolve to be tender with the young, compassionate with the aged, sympathetic with the striving, and tolerant with the weak and the wrong. Sometime in life you will have been all of these.**" Bob Goddard

SUFFERER,

You were not afraid to suffer for the greater good. Most great leaders have pushed through great resistance, suffering and being misunderstood while trying to accomplish something great. You are not afraid of pain. You suffer with us. We are not alone in the journey. I will do my best to try to understand other people's pain without judgement, knowing it could easily be me challenged with something similar. When people hurt, I will feel their hurt with them so they feel validated and human. When people receive a victory or a promotion, I will rejoice with them. Help me again and again to feel and see through Your heart and Your eyes. Give me words that bring peace to those in a season of suffering.

Love,
Your Child

John 11:35 *"Jesus wept."*

Romans 12:15 *"Rejoice with them that do rejoice, and weep with them that weep."*

"It is often hard to distinguish between the hard knocks in life and those of opportunity." Frederick Phillips

TAKETH AWAY,

I know You know what is best for me. I want my life to be lined up with Your will. Shut doors and open doors have equal importance. Sometimes we are blessed by the shut doors and the people You remove from our path for whatever reason. Sometimes the blessing is in what You choose to take away. I came into this world with nothing and will go out of this world with nothing. I will remain in healthy attachment to people and things, knowing being overly attached is a form of dependency and unhealthy. I give You the freedom to remove people or things out of my life as You please without being frustrated and angry with the process. The truth is that being too attached shows I feel I have ownership over whatever I am overly attached to. I have no ownership. You are the owner of all things and all people. They belong to You. Therefore You have every right to remove as You wish. You are the King and it is Your kingdom, not mine.

Love,
Your Child

John 1:21 *"And said, Naked came I out of my mother's womb, and naked shall I return hither: the Lord gave, and the Lord hath taken away; blessed be the name of the Lord."*

> "Never mistake knowledge for wisdom. One helps you make a living; the other helps you make a life." Sandra Carey

REWARDER,

When I pray in secret, You reward by showing up for me in public. If what I am praying for does not line up to Your will for my life or bring You glory, then I pray You do not answer the prayer my way. I know anything is possible. You can change a situation any time You want. I gain wisdom from my experiences in this life. Some are good and some are bad. Wisdom is my reward for experience. I will continue on my journey and share the wisdom I have learned with others in hopes that they will not have to suffer through some of the same painful choices I made in order to receive the wisdom I received through experience.

Love,
Your Child

Mathew 6:2 *"Therefore when thou doest thine alms, do not sound a trumpet before thee, as the hypocrites do in the synagogues and in the streets, that they may have glory of men. Verily I say unto you, They have their reward."*

James 4:3 *"Ye ask, and receive not, because ye ask amiss, that ye may consume it upon your lusts."*

Hebrews 11:6 *"But without faith, it is impossible to please him: for he that cometh to God must believe that he is a rewarder of them that diligently seek him."*

> "The most dangerous untruths are truths moderately distorted."
> George Christoph Lichtenburg

BUILDER,

Your Word is my foundation. I need to know as much of it as I can so that I will be strong in You. Help me to speak the truth at all times. I choose to trust in Your Word above all else. I enjoy reading, learning and comparing other Bible versions to the original to receive a better understanding; however, I will pay attention and acknowledge if other versions of Your Word "take away" or "add to" certain parts of the original meaning. I always compare to make sure other versions line up with the original English text, the King James Version, which is the closest translation to the original Hebrew and Greek words. I need to be a person of my word like You are a person of Your Word. Let me not exaggerate the truth nor portray myself falsely to impress others. Exaggerations are lies and not truths. Honesty and trust is required to have a strong foundation in You and a strong foundation in all of my other relationships.

Love,
Your Child

Ephesians 4:29 *"Let no corrupt communication proceed out of your mouth, but that which is good to the use of edifying, that it may minister grace unto the hearers."*

Hebrews 11:10 *"For he looked for a city which hath foundations, whose builder and maker is God."*

> "The greatest gift you can give another is the purity of your attention."
> Richard Moss, MD

LISTENER,

You hear me any time of the day or of the night. I do not have to make an appointment to talk with You. Sometimes I hear You talk back to me with that still, small voice inside of my heart. Sometimes You talk back to me through a person. Sometimes You choose to talk back to me through Your Word. Help me to act on whatever You speak to me to do. You are always available to talk with. You hear what I am not saying. You read between the lines. You know my intentions and understand the feelings behind my words. You are the greatest listener. I want to be able to listen to others the way You intensely listen to me. I want to listen to others the way I want to be listened to. If I notice someone is struggling listening to me talk, let me not take it personal. It could be that they have a condition that hinders their listening skills, such as ADHD, autism, or maybe they are having side effects to a medication that is hindering their attention span. I will give grace the way I would want grace.

Love,
Your Child

Romans 2:13 *"For not the hearers of the law are just before God, but the doers of the law shall be justified."*

"Boredom is a vital problem for the moralist, since at least half the sins of mankind are caused by the fear of it."

JUDGE,

Your Word judges me. I know right from wrong in Your eyes when I read Your Word. Help me to confront sin in my life and be proactive about stopping sin in my life. I do not want to justify sin in my life and make it "ok" to where I do not attempt to change, but instead accept the sin. Let me always be willing to put forth my best efforts in not willfully sinning. When I do sin, I will not mentally beat myself up, but instead accept Your forgiveness and take on an action plan on what I need to do to change. I also will not judge another's journey, which is between You and them. It is not my place to take on Your part in their life. I cannot "play God" in other people's lives to "teach them a lesson" or get them to do what I think they should be doing (unless I am parenting a child). You are the greatest teacher; You are the judge and You are God and do Your job well without my help. I will love people where they are at without trying to manipulatively control their them by attempting to play "Your Part" in their journey. I will trust You by putting the difficult people in my path in Your hands, knowing You are doing "Your Part" in their journey.

Love,
Your Child

Revelation 21:8 *"But the fearful, and unbelieving, and the abominable, and murders, and whoremongers, and sorcerers, and idolaters, and all liars, shall have their part in the lake which burneth with fire and brimstone: which is the second death."*

"The art of living consists in knowing which impulses to obey and which must be made to obey." Sydney J. Harris

LIFEGIVER,

You give life. I speak "life" into my blood, into my liver, into my bones, into my muscles, into my lungs, into my brain, into my heart and into my situation. You are not only a representation of natural life, but of spiritual life. My life is created by my choices, not by chance. You light up the dark areas of my life so that I can receive revelation of what needs to change in me, or around me to be a better me. You shine in these areas so that I have an opportunity to make things right!! While You are a beautiful light in my life, let me be a light to those who only know darkness. Let me be a light of truth, encouragement, mercy, purpose, change, trust, healing, edification, love. Let me stand out and be the difference.

Love,
Your Child

1 Peter 2:9-10 *"But ye are a chosen generation, a royal priesthood, an holy nation, a peculiar people; that ye should shew forth the praises of him who hath called you out of darkness into his marvelous light; which in time past were not a people, but are now the people of God: which had not obtained mercy, but now have obtained mercy."*

> "What do we live for if it is not to make life less difficult for each other?"
> — George Eliot

GRACE,

When I have undeserved favor from You, it is Your grace at work in my life. Sometimes I worry about my future. How will I deal with tragedy, sickness, death of a relationship? Who will take care of me when I cannot take care of myself? How will I handle the unknown or something I know will challenge my faith? I do know this: if I have You with me I can get through anything and trust You to get me through it. You are an "on-time" God, and know when to step in my life to help me. You place the right people in my path at the right time to be Your healing hands and feet for me. I will be Your healing hands and feet also for others. I can trust You will show up in some way and will not leave me hanging.

Love,
Your Child

Psalms 46:1 *"God is our refuge and strength, a very present help in trouble."*

II Corinthians 12:9 *"And he said unto me, my grace is sufficient for thee: for my strength is made perfect in weakness. Most gladly therefore will I rather glory in my infirmities, that the power of Christ may rest upon me."*

> "No winter lasts forever; no spring skips its turn." Hal Borland

PATH OF LIFE,

There are many different seasons that are necessary for me to go through in order for me to grow. All seasons are important. Summer, Fall, Winter and Spring have their place in the natural. So it is with the spiritual. Some seasons are full of blessings. Some are dry seasons where we tend to grow the most. Some seasons we are grieving. Some seasons are a time of testing our character. Sometimes the change of seasons is an adjustment to a shift toward something new and unknown. I will make time, not "try to find time," to do what is necessary for each season You place me in. Help me to accept each season You bring and be grateful for the lessons they offer.

Love,
Your Child

Ecclesiastes 3:1-8 *"To everything there is a season, and a time to every purpose under heaven: A time to be born, and a time to die; a time to plant, and a time to pluck up that which is planted; A time to kill, and a time to heal; a time to break down, and a time to build up; A time to weep, and a time to laugh; a time to mourn, and a time to dance; A time to cast away stones, and a time to gather stones together; a time to embrace, and a time to refrain from embracing; A time to get, and a time to lose; a time to keep, and a time to cast away; A time to send, and a time to sew; a time to keep silence, and a time to speak; A time to love, and a time to hate; a time of war, and a time of peace."*

> "I sought to hear the voice of God and climbed the topmost steeple, but God declared: 'Go down again—I dwell among the people.'" John Henry Newman

CHRIST,

You are the Messiah talked about in the Old Testament. You are the Most Anointed One. I know Your name is Jesus. You take on many forms or titles such as Father, Son, Holy Ghost, Creator, Savior, Friend. You loved us so much that You came down to earth in flesh and lived among us so You could understand our world in human form and fulfill Your plan of salvation. Even though You wear many hats, Your name is Jesus and You are One Lord.

Love,
Your Child

Deuteronomy 6:4 *"Hear, O Israel: The Lord our God is one Lord..."*

John 14:9 *"Jesus saith unto him, Have I been so long time with you, and yet hast thou not known me, Philip? He that hath seen me hath seen the Father; and how sayest thou then, show us the Father?"*

Ephesians 4:5 *"One Lord, one faith, one baptism..."*

"No one ever excused his way to success." David Del dotto

STABILITY,

You are stable and want me to be stable. To be stable I must not react right away to a stressful situation but thoughtfully think it through with a good response. To be stable, I must not allow my brain to dwell on negativity. To be stable, I must not judge other people or the future by the failures or difficult people of my past. Just because my last similar experience was not good does not necessarily mean it will repeat itself. To be stable, I must embrace my present situation for what it is and not be in denial of the truth of it, nor try to change the truth of it. To be stable, I must not be afraid when life throws a curve ball and I have a detour to make in my journey. To be stable, I must not put on masks to impress certain people. To be stable, I cannot take everything personally. To be stable, I cannot participate in risky activities that are dangerous. Help me to be a stable, balanced person.

Love,
Your Child

James 1:8 *"A double minded man is unstable in all his ways."*

"A truly great book should be read in youth, again in maturity and once more in old age, as a fine building should be seen by morning light, at noon and by moonlight." Robertson Davies

LAMP,

    Your Word is a lamp that lights up each step I make, each moment of everyday. I do not have to know Your whole plan for my life. I do not have to see the whole path to walk on it. I am not responsible for Your part in Your plan for my life. I am only responsible for doing my part the way it is supposed to be done. I can trust You with Your part and with the outcome. I can seek You alone for each step I take, trusting in Your leading. I also do not need to try to "play God" in other peoples' lives to get them to respond or do things the way I think they should. Manipulating people with guilt and fear is a form of selfish control. I can trust others are truly in Your trustworthy hands.

Love,
Your Child

Psalm 119:105 *"Thy word is a lamp unto my feet, and a light unto my path."*

> "Discernment is God's call to intercession, never to faultfinding."
> — Corrie ten Boom

CORRECTOR,

Help me to discern when the enemy is trying to destroy Your blueprints and plans for my life. The enemy can use personality conflicts, misunderstandings, gossip, greed, and the desire for power or position to hinder what You really want for me. The enemy will also try to use my personal failures against me to try to stop me from believing I can minister to others. Help me to do Your will no matter what. Remind me when I fail that it is Your blood that makes me right, not me. I will never be good enough to be used by You, but what You did on the Cross makes me good enough. Make the enemy who is trying to destroy me and my destiny, destroy himself. I pray God will reverse the curses I have placed on myself or others through poor choices or negative, destroying words.

Love,
Your Child

John 10:10 *"The thief cometh not, but for to steal, and to kill, and to destroy: I am come that they might have life, and that they might have it more abundantly."*

> "Our rabbi once said, 'God always answers our prayers, it's just that sometimes the answer is no.'" Barbara Feinstein

KEEPER OF US,

Let me have such a heart for people and for Your purpose that I will be willing to pray deeply with everything in me and fast for Your purpose to be fulfilled. I know prayer and fasting breaks strongholds in the spirit realm, releases Your power, and destroys the enemy and his tactics. There are many ways to fast such as the Daniel fast, media fast, total fast, sunrise to sunset fast and liquid fast. When You lead me to fast and pray for something specific, let me do it in the manner and at the time that You lead me, not my own timing and my own way.

Love,
Your Child

Esther 4:1-3 "When Mordecai perceived all that was done, Mordecai rent his clothes, and put on sackcloth with ashes, and went out into the midst of the city, and cried with a loud and a bitter cry; And came even before the king's gate: for none might enter into the kings gate clothed with sackcloth. And in every province, whithersoever the king's commandment and his decree came, there was great mourning among the Jews, and fasting, and weeping, and sackcloth and ashes."

Daniel 10:3 "I ate no pleasant bread, neither came flesh nor wine in my mouth, neither did I anoint myself at all, till three whole weeks were fulfilled."

> "Those persons who say they have never been jealous, what they mean is that they have never been in love." Gerald Brenan

JEALOUS,

I know You are a jealous God because of Your immense love for me. You do not want me to serve any other gods or have any idols. Anyone or anything can be an idol. I do not want to idolize anyone but You. Help me to remove whatever or whoever is taking Your rightful place in my life. Money, position, shopping, power, drugs, alcohol, a person, and food can all be idolized. Help me to stay balanced in every area of my life. Help me to prioritize my time correctly. Let me be aware when something or someone is trying to take Your place. I do not want anyone or anything to steal my time with You. The enemy wants to destroy my relationship with You by distracting me with anything that can become an idol. I refuse to let that happen to us.

Love,
Your Child

Exodus 34:14 *"For thou shalt worship no other god: for the Lord, whose name is Jealous, is a Jealous God."*

Proverbs 11:1 *"A false balance is abomination to the Lord: but a just weight is his delight."*

"A good example is like a bell that calls many to church." **Danish Proverb**

WITNESS,

Help me to be willing to confront the truth about myself so that I can work on myself. I know I do not have it all together. I fail in so many areas of my life daily. I do not want to be a stumbling block in the way of others growth. Help me not to ruin my witness by behaving poorly in public. Let my life lead people to You, not lead people away from You. Help me to see what needs to change in me. Let me not ignore or deny the truth about myself because ignoring or denying the truth does not change the truth.

Love,
Your Child

Ephesians 5:1-10 *"Be ye therefore followers of God, as dear children; And walk in love, as Christ also hath loved us, and hath given himself for us an offering and a sacrifice to God for a sweet smelling savour. But fornication, and all uncleanness, or covetousness, let it not be one named among you, as becometh saints; neither filthiness, nor foolish talking, nor jesting, which are not convenient: but rather giving of thanks. For this ye know, that no whoremonger, not unclean person, not covetous man, who is an idolater, hath any inheritance in the kingdom of Christ and of God. Let no man deceive you with vain words: for because of these things cometh the wrath of God upon the children of disobedience. Be not ye therefore partakers with them. For ye were sometimes darkness, but now are ye light in the Lord: walk as children of light."*

> "True love begins when nothing is looked for in return."
> — Antoine de Saint-Exupery

GIVER OF FREEDOM OF CHOICE,

    Thank You for looking past my failures, regrets, and hurts. Thank You for still seeing my potential and meeting my needs in spite of myself. Help me to example Your same unconditional love toward myself and everyone else. Love does not try to change someone to be who I want them to be. Love does not do something to create the reaction I want. Love is when I love people for who they really are, not the image in my head that I want them to be. Love sees past the faults of others and pays attention to their growth and potential. Love allows people to make their own choices whether I agree or disagree with their choices. Love gives people the freedom to live out their purpose without trying to stop them for my own selfish needs to be met.

Love,
Your Child

1 John 4:7-8 *"Beloved, let us love one another: for love is of God; and everyone that loveth is born of God, and knoweth God. He that loveth not knoweth not God; for God is love."*

> "If you can find a path with no obstacles, it probably doesn't lead anywhere."
> Frank A. Clark

GOD OF THE 2ND, 3RD, 4TH AND SO MANY CHANCES,

I refuse to give up because I know You have not given up on me. As long as I am breathing, hope for change will remain. Hope for healing, hope for deliverance, hope for reconciliation between me and others, hope for miracles, and hope for a continuing purpose.

Love,
Your Child

Psalms 71:14 *"But I will hope continually, and will yet praise thee more and more."*

"There are no secrets to success. It is the result of preparation, hard work, learning from failure." General Colin L. Powell

PREPARER,

I need favor with You and who You want me to have favor with so that I can fulfill Your will. Put the right people in my path both to help me and for me to help. Before making any decision, help me to pray about it and investigate everything about it first. Let me not be impulsive in making any decision until I know I have heard from You. Let me work hard at each step You reveal to me to prepare for the next step. Let me be committed to give the work You put in front of me my very best efforts. I know Your will is what is best for me. You know what I need and You know what I do not need. I would rather be in Your will than to be miserable in my will because my experience shows that my will was not what I thought it would be once it happened.

Love,
Your Child

Proverbs 24:27 "Prepare thy work without, and make it fit for thyself in the field; and afterward build thine house."

"Don't go on discussing what a good person should be. Just be one."
— Marcus Aurelius

JUST,

You crossed all boundaries to be there for people—race, cultural, religious and social status—when it was not popular to do so. You were way ahead of Your time while You were here on Earth. Help me to be the same person with everyone and treat everyone the same and justly. Let me not show favoritism one toward another for any reason.

Love,
Your Child

Acts 10:34 *"Then Peter opened his mouth, and said, of a truth I perceive that God is no respecter of persons."*

"I like people who are loyal to me, and I like to be loyal, too." George Strait

COURAGE,

I do not want to be one of those people who only lives for You when You are providing healing or performing miracles in my life. When You were in the form of Jesus, people were only there for You when You were popular. When it was time for You to bear our cross, most people disappeared. This was when You needed people the most. I want to be devoted to You whether it is raining or shining in my life. I want people to be there for me during both popular times and during my worst times. I pray that I can be loyal to You and others too.

Love,
Your Child

Isaiah 41:6 *"They helped everyone his neighbor; and everyone said to his brother, Be of good courage."*

"People want to know how much you care before they care how much you know." Theodore Roosevelt

CARING,

I do not ever want to be cliquish. I want to be able to mingle in any setting or group of people. I want all sorts of friends with different backgrounds and different interests. Let me make everyone around me feel comfortable and welcome. I want to put people at ease when they are nervous and trying to fit in.

Love,
Your Child

Colossians 3:12-13 *"Put on therefore, as the elect of God, holy and beloved, bowels of mercies, kindness, humbleness of mind, meekness, long suffering; For bearing on another, and forgiving one another, if any man have a quarrel against any; even as Christ forgave you, so also do ye."*

"Be cautious. Opportunity does the knocking for temptation too." Al Batt

RESCUER,

I know some people want to tempt me to do wrong things so that they can use it against me and assassinate my reputation. Help me to ignore temptation no matter what form it takes. Just because I have been set free from an addiction or sin does not mean I will not be tempted in it in the future! Help me to guard my heart, mind, and spirit. I also know that as I grow in my walk with You, temptations can change. Help me to put on the whole armor of God and to pay attention to Your way of escape. When I fall, help me to be aware of what my trigger was, so I can learn how to be a better warrior for my salvation and destiny. Let me forgive myself and not dwell on it, but choose to move forward. Rehashing my failures merely makes me feel worse and is toxic to my growth and present purpose.

Love,
Your Child

Ephesians 6:10-18 *"Finally, by brethren, be strong in the Lord, and in the power of his might. Put on the whole armour of God, that ye may be able to stand against the wiles of the devil. For we wrestle not against flesh and blood, but against principalities, against spiritual wickedness in high places. Wherefore take unto you the whole armour of God, that ye may be able to withstand in the evil day, and having done all, to stand. Stand therefore, having your lions girt about with truth, and having on the breastplate of righteousness; And your feet shod with the preparation of the gospel of peace; Above all, taking the shield of faith, wherewith ye shall be able to quench all the firery darts of the wicked. And take the helmet of salvation, and the sword of the Spirit, which is the word of God: Praying always with all prayer and supplication in the Spirit, and watching thereunto with all perseverance and supplication for all saints."*

"Accept me as I am – only then will we discover each other." Federico Fellini

My APPROVAL,

Let me not buy things to make me appear in a higher social status. Doing that is the desire for the approval of others. When I try to manipulate the way people view me, I am using their approval to feel better about myself, which really reveals my own lack of fulfillment. You approve me, not what I am wearing or the kind of car I drive or the home I live in. The Gospels tell me that in Your ministry on this earth, You reached out to everyone. You didn't care about what people thought. You love everyone without condition. You love the wealthy. You love the homeless. You love the socially unacceptable. You love the ones who committed all sorts of crimes. You love the mentally and physically ill. You love those who disagree with You. You love those who did You wrong purposely. I am convinced people see Your love through us when we treat everyone equally and when we forgive the inexcusable. You love and can use imperfect people.

Love,
Your Child

John 15:12 *"This is my commandment, that ye love one another, as I have loved you."*

> "When we are well, we all have good advice for those who are ill."
> Lucius Annaeus Seneca

ROCK,

I know Your ways do not always make sense to me all the time. It is easy for people to tell you what they think you should do about your problems when they are not living with the problem. Help me to trust You with the outcome of my prayer requests and my life. I do not want to get stuck on focusing on a present test or trial. You know the big picture and the bigger plan. So I will do my part by taking care of myself. I will be responsible for exercising, eating right, keeping my environment clean and organized, taking my medicine and vitamins, going to all doctor's appointments, resting when I need to, being a blessing to whoever comes in my path and trusting that You will do Your part. You are my Rock and my foundation; I will stand on Your promises.

Love,
Your Child

Isaiah 55:8 *"For my thoughts are not your thoughts, neither are your ways my ways, saith the Lord."*

"Manners are a sensitive awareness of the feelings of others. If you have that awareness, you have good manners, no matter what fork you use." Emily Post

AWARE,

    Help me to be aware of how I am affecting those around me. Do they feel better when I leave the room, or do they feel worse? Am I building people up with my words, or am I participating in assassinating the character of others with my words? I want to protect people's reputations. Am I draining people's energy and spirits by complaining about my problems? Am I paying attention to their needs while with them? Help me to be more aware of how I am affecting Your world and furthering Your kingdom.

Love,
Your Child

Hebrews 13:2 *"Be not forgetful to entertain strangers; for thereby some have entertained angels unaware."*

> "You do not lead by hitting people over the head. That's assault, not leadership."
> Dwight D. Eisenhower

LEADER,

Making amends is so important. Also confessing my wrongs is very important. When I admit my failures, I rob them of their power over me. I do not want anything to have power over me except Your Spirit, Your Word and Your Love that not only changes me but leads me in my journey. I want You to be my leader, not a person, not a substance, not power, not wealth, not my desires but Your desires for me. I submit myself to Your Leadership. If I am put in any leadership position, let me not abuse others verbally, be controlling, belittle others under me or get a "big head" over a position. I pray to allow others to help and work as a good team player. Everyone deserves to feel a part of the group. I know You can remove me at any time if I take advantage of a position.

Love,
Your Child

James 5:16 *"Confess your faults one to another, and pray one for another, that ye may be healed. The effectual fervent prayer of a righteous man availeth much."*

"Money is a good servant but a bad master." French Proverb

GIVER,

Help me to be wise in my finances. Let me pay my bills on time. Let me always put something aside for savings. Let me invest in my future. Let me be a cheerful giver, giving to others as You would lead me. Everything that I have is not mine; it belongs to You. I am not emotionally attached to any of my possessions. Let me know when to say "yes," and when to say "no" to others when they ask for my support financially. I know I only receive so that I can give. At the same time, I do not want to get in the way of the financial lessons You are trying to teach someone by enabling them with my giving. Let me give only as You see fit.

Love,
Your Child

Luke 6:38 *"Give, and it shall be given unto you; good measure, pressed down, and shaken together, and running over, shall men give into your bosom. For with the same measure that ye mete withal it shall be measured to you again."*

Day 122

"For the strength of the Pack is the Wolf, and the strength of the Wolf is the Pack." Rudyard Kipling

PEACE SPEAKER,

Help me to be in unity with my family, church, job and doctors. Let me be a team player, focused on the ultimate purpose of why we do what we do and not get caught up in personality conflicts, disagreements, gossip, or anything that can hinder all of us from fulfilling the ultimate goal together as a team. When something goes wrong in the group, let me be the one who brings people together and creates peace like You do. Help me to forgive quickly and to not take anything personally, but to be easy to be around and work with, always staying focused on the goal.

Love,
Your Child

Proverbs 6:14-19 *"Frowardness is in his heart, he deviseth mischief continually; he soweth discord. Therefore shall his calamity come suddenly; suddenly shall he be broken without remedy. These six things doth the Lord hate: yea, seven are an abomination unto him: A proud look, a lying tongue, and hands that shed innocent blood, An heart that deviseth wicked imaginations, feet that be swift in running to mischief, A false witness that speaketh lies, and he that soweth discord among brethren."*

"The ultimate measure of a man is not where he stands in moments of comfort and convenience, but where he stands at times of challenge and controversy."
Martin Luther King, Jr.

RESURRECTION,

    Your power that raised Christ up from the dead lives in me and empowers me to do what I am called to do. It empowers me to get and maintain the power over any sin trying to dominate my life. It empowers me to be the best me I can be. It empowers me to live healthily and do what I need to do to stay healthy. It empowers me to adjust myself to the changing of seasons in my life. It empowers me to stand up for the underdog and to stand up for what is right. It empowers me to say "no" when I want to say "yes." It empowers me to live and not die. Therefore, it is important I connect with You daily so I can have the power I need to get through each day.

Love,
Your Child

Micah 7:8 *"Rejoice not against me, O mine enemy: when I fall, I shall arise; when I sit in darkness the Lord shall be a light unto me."*

> "You must be willing to protect yourself and what you cherish, no matter what the cost." Christopher Paolini

PROTECTOR,

    I pray to be under the umbrella of Your protection. I plead the blood of Jesus over my mind, body and spirit. I pray for traveling mercies when going anywhere throughout my day. I pray a hedge of protection around about me to protect me from anyone or anything You have not ordained to be in my path. I pray against any spirit not of You that may try to influence me or attach itself to me. Your blood covering me and my life is the greatest protection I have. When I speak for You, hide me under Your blood, let people not see me, but let them see You at work through me. Let them not be focused on me as the messenger, but to be focused only on the message I am to give them for You.

Love,
Your Child

Proverbs 4:23 *"Keep thy heart with all diligence; for out of it are the issues of life."*

> "Worry is like a rocking chair. It will give you something to do but won't get you anywhere." The United Church Observer

SOUND MIND,

Sometimes I tend to over-think things. I want to make sure I am looking at the facts, not what I think happened. Help me to not create scenarios in my head out of my fears. Give me a mind that has clarity and looks for the best instead of assuming the worst first. I choose to trust You with the outcome. I choose to give people the benefit of the doubt. Take away the worries and fears that try to dominate my mind over my decisions. I know not to make a decision based on an unhealthy fear. I also do not want to make decisions based on past failures. Just because I failed at something in the past does not mean I will fail at it in the future.

Love,
Your Child

2 Timothy 1:7 *"For God, hath not given us the spirit of fear; but of power, and of love, and of a sound mind."*

"To have a successful team every player must want the same thing and dream the same dream." Luke John Daly

FORBEARING ONE ANOTHER,

    I know I cannot be the perfect employee every day, and I know not to put unrealistic expectations on those around me. Let me not have a reputation of only confronting what is going wrong on the job, but always see the good in what people are doing. If someone is having a bad day or not feeling well, let me be a team player and not only do my job, but help them with theirs. After all, I would want someone to do the same for me.

Love,
Your Child

I Corinthians 12:14 *"For the body is not one member, but many."*

"Character is what you know you are, not what others think you are."
Marva Collins and Civia Tamarkin

UPRIGHT,

If being true to who I think that I am permits any sin in my life, or living in a way contrary to Your Word, then I do not want to be true to who I am. I cannot use this as an excuse to live how I please. I want to be true to who Your Word says I am. I have to change my life to live up to Your principles, not change Your Word to fit the life I want to have. So place the desire in me to be who I am supposed to be for You.

Love,
Your Child

Psalms 15:1-2 *"Lord, who shall abide in thy tabernacle? who shall dwell in thy holy hill? He that walketh uprightly, and speaketh the truth in his heart."*

"If you can find a path with no obstacles, it probably doesn't lead anywhere."
Frank A. Clark

DILIGENT,

Help me not to dwell on things that happened in the past. I do not live there anymore. I want to live in the present, enjoying each moment as it is given to me. I do not want to waste time over things I cannot do anything about. I choose to stay focused on moving toward my goals. I want to stay focused on making each moment I am alive as productive as it can be.

Love,
Your Child

Philippians 3:13-14 *"Brethren, I count not myself to have apprehended; but this one thing I do, forgetting those things which are behind, and reaching forth unto those things which are before. I press toward the mark for the prize of the high calling of God in Christ Jesus."*

> "Honesty and transparency make you vulnerable.
> Be honest and transparent anyways." Mother Theresa

REAL,

Help me to not feel as though I have to change according to who I am around. I do not have to live life wearing masks. I do not have to be the perfect person, mentor, worker, friend, or family member. I can accept my humanity with its flaws and illnesses. I can be comfortable with who You created me to be. There is no need to live a life of trying to prove myself to anyone. Who I am in You is enough.

Love,
Your Child

1 Thessalonians 4:1 *"Furthermore then we beseech you, brethren, and exhort you by the Lord Jesus, that as ye have received of us how ye ought to walk and to please God, so ye would abound more and more."*

"Temptation rarely comes in working hours. It is in their leisure time that men are made or marred." W.N. Taylor

GOD,

When I am bored or lonely, help me to not make self-destructive decisions that could damage my future. It is normal to have down time. Let me use my down time to do good things for myself. I know You always promise a way to deal with temptation. Let me not be impulsive doing only what my emotions lead me to do; I cannot be controlled by my emotions. I need to make my decisions based on what is right, not how I feel. Let my decisions be informed and fully thought out. Wrong decisions can lead to guilt, regret and depression. It is not worth it. Let my decisions please You.

Love,
Your Child

1 Corinthians 10:13 *"There hath no temptation taken you but such as is common to man: but God is faithful who will not suffer you to be tempted above that ye are able; but will with the temptation also make a way to escape, that ye may be able to bear it."*

"Real joy comes not from ease or riches or from the praise of men, but from doing something worthwhile." Sir Wilfred Grenfell

RICHES,

I found riches when I found You. True riches are salvation, peace of mind, helping others grow and joyful times with family and friends. I am more interested in quality of life with You than earthly riches. How I spend my time means more to me than anything. True riches is doing what is right when it is easier to do what is wrong. I consider myself very rich, not because of material or financial gain, but because I have the greatest relationship with "The Greatest One of All." You make me rich. So I seek You, Your Presence, Your Guidance. I fill myself up with Your love so I can pour it out to everyone around me. Thank You for making me rich with You and Your Great Principles!

Love,
Your Child

Matthew 6:19-21"Lay not up for yourselves treasures upon earth, where moth and rust doth corrupt, and where thieves break through and steal: But lay up for yourselves treasures in heaven, where neither moth nor rust doth corrupt, and where thieves do not break through nor steal: For where your treasure is, there will your heart be also."

"That's the secret of entertaining. You make your guests feel welcome and at home. If you do that honestly, the rest takes care of itself." Barbara Hall

HOSPITALITY,

Help me to be more sensitive to the needs of those around me. Help me to meet the need if I can. If someone is sick with the flu, I can drop off homemade soup to them. If someone is grieving, I can send a card letting them know they are thought of. If I have guests over, I can make sure they feel welcome and comfortable. If someone needs to talk, I can stop everything I am doing, keep eye contact with them and listen. If someone is bed ridden, I can run errands for them. If someone has no transportation, I can help them with a ride every now and then.

Love,
Your Child

Matthew 25:21 "His lord said unto him, Well done, thou good and faithful servant: thou hast been faithful over a few things, I will make thee ruler over many things: enter thou into the joy of thy lord."

Mathew 25:40 "And the King shall answer and say unto them, Verily I say unto you, Inasmuch as he have done it unto one of the least of these my brethren, he have done it unto me."

> "If you spend your time talking to God about everything, you'll be less likely to vent your feelings to everyone." Buky Ojelabi

BELOVED,

No one knows me like You do. You know everything about me, even the number of hairs on my head. Help me to be careful about how much I use people as a sounding board. The more I talk about the problem, the more power I give it in my life. Help me to pray about it, feel the feelings, release it and then actively choose to move on from it. I don't want life's problems to ruin a whole day for me. Everyone has problems and we have to encourage each other, not discourage each other by talking about the problem too much.

Love,
Your Child

Mathew 10:30 *"But the very hairs of your head are all numbered."*

Matthew 11:28-30 *"Come unto me, all ye that labour and are heavy laden, and I will give you rest. Take my yoke upon you, and learn of me; for I am meek and lowly in heart: and ye shall find rest unto your souls. For my yoke is easy, and my burden is light."*

"I gave myself permission to be imperfect a long time ago." Rebecca Boyett

RIGHTEOUS,

You are my righteousness. I know everything was created for Your Glory. Our failures keep us humble. It also keeps people from idolizing us. You are the only perfect one. It was never Your intention for anyone to be worshiped. I do not want my world to revolve around a person. I want my world to revolve around You and make this world a better place. What You did on the Cross is how I am qualified to do Your work. Thank You for Your blood that makes me clean. When I am being used by You in any form, let people not see me, but let them see You at work through me. All I am is an imperfect messenger delivering the perfect message.

Love,
Your Child

Isaiah 64:6 "But we are all as an unclean thing, and all our righteousness are as filthy rags; and our iniquities, like the wind, have taken us away."

II Corinthians 12:6-7 "For though I would desire to glory, I shall not be a fool; but now I forbear, lest any man should think of me above that which he seeth me to be, or that he heareth of me. And lest I should be exalted above measure through the abundance of the revelations, there was given to me a thorn in the flesh, the messenger of Satan to buffet me, lest I should be exalted above measure.

> "Voices that loud are always meant to bully. Do not be bullied. Acts of bravery don't always take place on battlefields. They can take place in your heart, when you have the courage to honor your character, your intellect, your inclinations, and yes, your soul by listening to its clean, clear voice of direction instead of following the muddied messages of a timid world."
>
> Anna Quindlen

RADICAL,

Sometimes you have to take a costly risk to accomplish something. I refuse to live with unnecessary regrets out of fear that something will not work out. I won't choose not to try out of fear of failure or fear of rejection. You give me the confidence it takes to be bold and courageous with my choices. You enable me to stand up for what is right. You grant me the ability to do what I thought was impossible. Your power working in me enables me to accomplish the impossible. So I will choose to take risks that can challenge my reputation. I believe in You and Your cause enough to walk into my purpose with no fear!

Love,
Your Child

Luke 12:11-12 "And when they bring you unto the synagogues, and unto magistrates, and powers, take ye no thought how or what thing ye shall answer, or what ye shall say: For the Holy Ghost shall teach you in the same hour what ye ought to say."

> "Man must evolve for all human conflict a method which rejects revenge, aggressions and retaliation. The foundation of such a method is love."
>
> Martin Luther King, Jr.

PRINCE OF PEACE,

I know I can come to a place of acceptance over things in my life. Things may have happened to me that I know were unfair. I do not have to allow my hurts or my failures to define me. I can make peace with the things I do not understand. I can forgive, let go and move forward without giving my past mistakes and present mistakes the power to affect my future. I know it is alright to feel upset and angry when a memory pops up. It is not acceptable to take it out on people around me, nor is it acceptable to make self-destructive choices because of it. Revenge is not an option.

Love,
Your Child

Romans 12:17-21 *"Recompense to no man evil for evil. Provide things honest in the sight of all men. If it be possible, as much as lieth in you, live peaceably with all men. Dearly beloved, avenge not yourselves, but rather give place unto wrath: for it is written, Vengeance is mine; I will repay, saith the Lord. Therefore if thine enemy hunger, feed him; if he thirst, give him drink: for in so doing thou shalt heap coals of fire on his head. Be not overcome of evil, but overcome evil with good."*

"All truths are easy to understand once they are discovered; the point is to discover them." Galileo Galilei

LORD OF LORDS,

I know that every scripture matters and counts. It is all inspired by You. I cannot pick and choose what I want to apply to my life. I also have to rightly divide it, not making a judgment on one scripture, but look at all other scriptures connected to it in order to get the full meaning of what You are trying to say to me when I am reading it.

Love,
Your Child

II Timothy 2:15 *"Study to shew thyself approved unto God, a workman that needeth not to be ashamed, rightly dividing the word of truth."*

II Timothy 3:16 *"All scripture is given by inspiration of God, and is profitable for doctrine, for reproof, for correction, for instruction in righteousness..."*

"Dedication is writing your name on the bottom of a blank sheet of paper and handing it to the Lord for Him to fill in." Rick Renner

TRUSTWORTHY,

I know it is alright to bargain with You because Abraham did it when praying for Sodom and Gomorrah. When dealing with a helpless situation, I want to change Your mind immediately on the matter. Bargaining gives me a sense of control over my painful circumstances. It gives me hope that the situation may change. It is a defense mechanism when dealing with a harsh reality. Even if it does not change, at least I can say I did all I could do to change the situation. So I live with no regret. Regardless of the outcome, I trust You are in control and can help me deal with any circumstance, whether it goes away or not.

Love,
Your Child

Genesis 18:22-33 *"And the men turned their faces from thence, and went toward Sodom; but Abraham stood ye before the Lord. And Abraham drew near and said, Wilt thou also destroy the righteous with the wicked? Peradventure there be fifty righteous within the city: wilt thou also destroy and not spare the place for the fifty righteous that are therein? That be far from thee to do after this manner, to slay the righteous with the wicked; and that the righteous should be as the wicked, that be far from thee; Shall not the Judge of all the earth do right? And the Lord said, If I find in Sodom fifty righteous within the city, then I will spare all the place for their sakes. And Abraham answered and said, Behold now, I have taken upon me to speak unto the Lord, which am but dust and ashes: Peradventure there shall lack five of the fifty righteous: wilt thou destroy all the city for lack of five? And he said, If I find there forty and five, I will not destroy it. And he spake unto him yet again, and said, Peradventure there shall be forty found there. And he said, I will not do it for forty's sake. And he said unto him, Oh let not the Lord be angry, and I will speak: Peradventure there shall thirty be found there. And he said, I will not do it, if I find thirty there. And he said, Behold now, I have taken upon me to speak unto the Lord: Peradventure there shall be twenty found there. And he said, I will not destroy it for twenty's sake. And he said, Oh let not the Lord be angry, and I will speak yet but this one: Peradventure ten shall be found there. And he said, I will not destroy it for ten's sake. And the Lord went his way, as soon as he had left communing with Abraham: and Abraham returned unto his place.*

"To love is a glimpse of Heaven." Karen Sunde

HEAVEN,

I know that when I get to Heaven that there will be no sickness and sorrow. In Heaven, there will be no loneliness, no worries, no confusion, no questions, no anger, no doubts, no resentment and no hurt. It sounds like a perfect place and my mind has trouble imagining what it will be like. There will be peace, joy, love and acceptance! I know when my time comes to transition there that I will have completed the tasks You wanted me to fulfill. But most importantly, I will finally get to meet You! In the meantime while I am still here on Earth, help me to understand life will not be perfect because I am not in Heaven yet. Thank You for such a wonderful opportunity You created for Your people!

Love,
Your Child

Matthew 7:21 *"Not everyone that saith unto me, Lord, Lord shall enter into the Kingdom of heaven; but he that doeth the will of my Father is in Heaven."*

Health Awareness

Part Two

Health Awareness

God is The Ultimate Solution who has provided many solutions on earth for us to access to live the best we can. It is important for us to educate ourselves on whatever issues we and our loved ones may experience. Education is a method of healing. This is a brief informational description of some of the health and social issues people face.

For more information, please go to: **www.CDC.gov**

ADHD: Attention Deficit Hyperactive Disorder.
   Symptoms: *hyperactivity, struggles with paying attention, easily distracted, impulsive behaviors*
   Solution: *Medication and Behavior Therapy*

ADDICTION: *Regular dependentcy on a person, thing or substance to survive. Addiction is a disease in the brain in which the body adapts to the addiction and requires more of it. It is a big sign you might have a problem with addiction if you try to stop a behavior and cannot.*
   Symptoms: *Abnormal cravings that affect your life in a negative way, lying and hiding to maintain the problem, stealing, doing things you never thought you would do to keep up the addiction, work and relationship problems, legal problems, needing more and more of the addiction to feel fulfilled.*
   Solution: *12 Step Programs and Counseling*

ALZHEIMERS: *A progressive disease that causes the brain to slowly deteriorate.*
   Symptoms: *Problems with memory and thinking, confusion.*
   Solution: *Medications that can improve the communication process between the neurons, synapses and neurotransmitters in the brain*

ANOREXIA: *Obsession with losing weight and body image. Misperception of how they look rooted in fear and self-esteem.*
   Signs: *Abnormal dieting, abnormal exercising, irregular menstruation for women, problems with teeth, living a secret life of lying and hiding to maintain the problem, anemia, dry skin*
   Solution: *Counseling and in extreme cases, Hospitalization*

AUTISM: *A disorder that hinders a person's communication skills.*
   Symptoms: *Struggles with understanding and expressing feelings, overly sensitive, repetitive behaviors*
   Solution: *Medications and Therapy*

BIPOLAR DISORDER: *A mental condition where someone has unpredictable mood swings between mania and depression.*
   Symptoms: *Depression, inflated self-esteem, racing thoughts, grandiose thinking, participating in risky and self-destructive behaviors, leaving projects unfinished, sleeping problems*
   Solution: *Mood-Stabilizing Medications*

BONE CANCER: *This is a cancer in the bone. It is usually in the arms and legs.*
   Symptoms: *Pain in the bone, swelling and fractions*
   Solution: *Get tested immediately, surgery, radiation and chemotherapy*

BRAIN ANEURYSMS: *A blood vessel in the brain erupts and can cause a stroke.*
   Symptoms: *Extremely repetitive and painful headaches, vision problems, nausea and vomiting*
   Solution: *Repair the blood vessel by clipping and, or coiling*

BULIMIA: *When a person overeats by binging, then purges the food by forcing themselves to vomit, or by over-exercise. It is caused by low self-esteem and rooted in fear. This person has a distorted body image.*
   Signs: *Exercising too much, always going to the bathroom after eating, missing food in the house, regular use of laxatives, defensiveness when asked about weight and eating habits, never gains weight, a secret life of hiding and lying to maintain the problem*
   Solution: *Counseling, and in extreme cases, Hospitalization*

CHRONIC FATIGUE SYNDROME: *A disorder where someone is constantly exhausted no matter how much rest they get.*
   Symptoms: *Abnormal exhaustion. Too tired to get things done and have a productive day.*
   Solution: *An exercise plan. If there is any pain in the body then it needs to be controlled and managed. See a Specialist*

CODEPENDENCY: *When one person does what another person is able to do for themselves. An abnormal reliance on someone else. An enmeshed relationship. When you lose yourself in someone else, when your life revolves around keeping someone in your life. These people have been abused or neglected in some way by caretakers in childhood and look for love from difficult people because the caretakers in childhood were difficult.*
   Signs: *Staying in an unhealthy relationship to avoid being alone, enabling a person's unhealthy behaviors including substance abuse, clinginess, jealousy when the person you are attached to spends time with someone else, looking for reasons to stay in the relationship, sacrificing your own needs to meet someone else's needs, neglecting the other people placed in your life*
   Solution: *Detach from the one you are dependent on, set boundaries, spend time with others in a balanced way*

CROHN'S: *A bowel disease that causes inflammation of the intestinal tract.*
   Symptoms: *Anemia, weight loss, anal fissures, fatigue, abdominal pain, diarrhea*
   Solution: *Medications to prevent inflammation and Surgery*

DEPRESSION: *When someone has extreme sadness that hinders their work life and relationships.*
   Symptoms: *A negative perception on everything, uncontrollable bouts of crying, isolating from others, sleep problems, a loss of interest in activities that are normally enjoyed*
   Solution: *Get out of yourself and help someone else. Make a list of what you are grateful for. Stay active in life. Counseling and Antidepressants*

DOMESTIC VIOLENCE: *Abusive behavior within the home, often physical violence.*
   Signs: *Physical harm, including but not limited to pushing, punching, beating, throwing across a room, destroying personal items, forcing others to drink or use drugs as a method of control, sexual abuse, emotional abuse.*
   Solution: *If it is an emergency then call the police immediately, get help, go to a shelter, get involved in a support group to heal, hospitalization*

EMOTIONAL ABUSE: *Abusive behavior involved in controlling other's emotions*
   Signs: *Belittling, shaming someone for their weaknesses or failures in front of a group of people, verbal abuse, sexual abuse, physical violence, extreme jealousy, manipulative threats to get you to do what they want, emotional blackmail, not allowing you the freedom to make your own decisions, accusing you of doing wrong with no facts to back it up*
   Solution: *If it is an emergency then call the police immediately, get help, go to a shelter, get involved in a support group to heal*

EPILEPSY: *A neurological disorder of abnormal electrical activity in the brain.*
   Symptom: *Seizures*
   Solution: *Anticonvulsant Medications*

FRAGILE X: *A genetic disorder characterized by learning disabilities.*
   Symptoms: *Problems with intellectual learning, narrow face and large ears, trouble with speech, problems understanding social interactions, bothered by certain sensations*
   Solution: *Medications and Therapy*

HEART DISEASE: *A cardiovascular disease.*
   Symptoms: *Sweating, dizziness, weakness, shortness of breath, discomfort in the chest area, irregular pulse, swelling in the ankles and feet*
   Solution: *Stent Placement, Heart Bypass Surgery, Medications, Quit Smoking, Exercise Daily, Eat Healthy, Rest Well, Maintain a Healthy Weight, Get checked regularly*

HIV: *Human Immunodeficiency Virus that can lead to AIDS (Acquired Immunodeficiency Syndrome). It is an immune system disease where the immune system struggles with fighting infections. HIV is caused by unprotected sexual behaviors and dirty needles. It is caught by contact with infected blood.*
   Symptoms: *Repetitive cough, swollen lymph nodes, high fever, weight loss, flu-like symptoms, fatigue*
   Solution: *If you know you have put yourself at risk then get tested for HIV. Use protection when intimate. Take medication right away, exactly as prescribed. Stay away from stressful situations, practice healthy habits.*

HUMAN TRAFFICKING: *Anytime a person is sold for sexual activity, whether it be forced sex slavery, prostitution for drugs or money, stripping in clubs.*
   Ways People Lure Others Into Being Trafficked: *Promising a hopeful future to someone who comes from a troubled home or who is homeless. If the person being lured uses substances and has an addiction already, then they promise an unlimited supply of that substance. Once they offer the substance for free over a period of time to the point where a person is becoming more dependent on the substance, then they withhold the substance as a means of control and begin to prostitute the victim out without providing enough of the addictive substance the body craves, and without allowing the victim to keep the money paid from the sex act. They look for people who are struggling finding a job, for young people who are vulnerable with low self-esteem, who are looking for love and acceptance. They promise great opportunities for the future.*
   Solution: *Talk to and educate others around you so they are not easily manipulated. If you are being trafficked then get help immediately. Get away from everyone keeping you in that life; go to shelter in another city or area. Get counseling for healing of incidents that took place.*

LUPUS: *When the immune system attacks its own tissues. It is an inflammatory disease.*
   Symptoms: *anemia, abnormal fatigue, swollen joints, fever*
   Solution: *Get tested for it, Medications*

MUSCULAR DYSTROPHY (MD): *A genetic disorder that weakens the muscles.*
  Symptoms: *Falling a lot, waddling gait, muscle pain, difficulty getting up or lying down or sitting, struggling with running or jumping, walks on the toes, large calf muscles*
  Solution: *Get a Muscle Biopsy, Medications and Therapy*

MEDULOBLASTOMA: *This is a cancerous brain tumor that is in the back bottom area of the skull. The cancer can spread to other parts of the body.*
  Symptoms: *Trouble with handwriting, vision problems, clumsiness, headaches, drowsiness, appetite changes*
  Solution: *Surgery to remove the tumor, chemotherapy, radiation, stem cell transplant*

OBESITY: *Abnormal overweight. It can shorten someone's lifespan and lead to health conditions such as diabetes and heart disease.*
  Sign: *Extreme Excessive Weight*
  Solution: *Get tested and find out if you have a medical condition that may be causing the extra weight and making it difficult to lose weight, eat healthy, exercise*

POST TRAUMATIC STRESS DISORDER (PTSD): *Usually caused from experiencing extreme trauma. War veterans and abuse victims tend to have this disorder.*
  Signs: *Avoidance of places that remind you of the trauma, nightmares, angry or aggressive outbursts, substance abuse to cope with memories, flashbacks, sleeping problems, difficulty in maintaining close relationships*
  Solution: *Therapy, Medications and Counseling*

SEXUALLY TRANSMITTED DISEASES (STDs): *Sexually transmitted diseases caused from being unprotected while being intimate with someone who is infected. Herpes, gonorrhea, HIV/AIDS, chlamydia, genital warts, syphilis, trichomoniasis*
  Symptoms: *Symptoms are not always obvious, and sometimes do not show up until it is too late, if you know you have put yourself at risk then you need to get tested, if you have been sexually active then you are at risk because at times even using protection does not help*
  Solution: *Get tested for everything right away if you know you are at risk*

SUICIDE: *When someone ends their own life. It is caused by extreme depression and other factors. If you or someone in your path desire to end life, get help immediately.*
   Symptoms: *Extreme depression, isolation from others, substance abuse to cope with emotional pain, looking for ways to end life, talk of being a burden to other people,*
   Solution: *Get Help Immediately, Counseling, Medications*

ULCERATIVE COLITIS: *An inflammatory bowel disease that causes ulcers and inflammation in the digestive tract.*
   Symptoms: *Anal bleeding, constant urgency to use the restroom, fatigue, weight loss, diarrhea with pus or blood in it, abdominal pain, problems using the restroom.*
   Solution: *Change in eating habits, Medications, Surgery to have an ostomy bag to hold waste*

Healing Scriptures

Part Three

Healing Scriptures

All Scriptures are from the King James Version of the Holy Bible.

Romans 10:17 *"So then faith cometh by hearing, and hearing by the Word of God."*

Jeremiah 30:17 *"For I will RESTORE Health unto thee, and I will heal thee of thy wounds, saith the Lord….."*

Mathew 18:19 *"Again I say unto you, that if two of you shall agree on earth as touching anything that they shall ask, it shall be done for them of my Father which is in Heaven. For where two or three are gathered together in my name, there am I in the midst of them."*

Jeremiah 17:14 *"Heal me O Lord, and I shall be healed; save me, and I shall be saved: for thou art my praise."*

Mark 9:24 *"And straightway the father of the child cried out, and said with tears, Lord, I believe; help thou mine unbelief."*

Mathew 15:28 *"Then Jesus answered and said unto her, O woman, great is thy faith: be it unto thee as thou wilt. And her daughter was made whole from that very hour."*

Psalms 40:10 *"I have not hid thy righteousness within my heart; I have declared thy faithfulness and thy salvation: I have not concealed thy loving kindness and thy truth from the great congregation."*

Mathew 9:22 *"But Jesus turned about, and when he saw her, he said, Daughter, be of good comfort, thy faith hath made thee whole. And the woman was made whole from that hour."*

Acts 4:22 *"For the man was above 40 years old, on who, this miracle of healing shewed."*

Mathew 9:35 *"And Jesus went about all the cities and villages, teachings in their synagogues, and preaching the gospel of the kingdom, and healing every sickness and every disease among the people."*

Mark 4:39-40 *"And he arose, and rebuked the wind, and said unto the sea, Peace, be still. And the wind ceased, and there was a great calm. And he said unto them, why are ye so fearful? How is it that we have no faith?"*

Mathew 17:20-21 *"And Jesus said unto them, because of your unbelief: for verily I say unto you, if ye have fight as a grain of mustard seed, we shall say unto this mountain, remove hence to yonder place: and it shall remove; and nothing shall be impossible unto you. Howbeit this kind goeth not out but by prayer and fasting."*

Jeremiah 32:27 *"Behold, I am the Lord, The God of all Flesh: is there anything too hard for me?"*

John 10:27 *"My sheep hear my voice, and I know them, and they follow me."*

Ruth 4:15 *"And he shall be unto thee a restorer of thy life, and a nourisher of thine old age . . ."*

John 3:2 *"The same came to Jesus by night, and said unto him, Rabbi, we know that thou art a teacher come from God: for no man can do these miracles that thou doest, except God be with Him."*

Psalms 143:1 *"Hear my prayer O Lord, give ear to my supplications: in thy faithfulness answer me, and in thy righteousness."*

Deuteronomy 7:9 *"Know therefore that the Lord thy God, he is God, the faithful God, which keepeth covenant and mercy with them that love him and keep his commandments to a thousand generations."*

Mathew 21:21 *"Jesus answered and said unto them, verily I say unto you, if ye have faith, and doubt not, ye shall not only do this which is done to the fig tree, but also if ye shall say unto this mountain, be thou removed, and be thou cast unto the sea; it shall be done."*

Mathew 9:29 *"Then he touched their eyes, saying, According to your faith be it unto you."*

Mark 5:34 *"And he said unto her, Daughter, thy faith hath made thee whole; go in peace, and be whole of thy plague."*

Psalms 89:1 *"I will sing of the mercies of the Lord forever: with my mouth will I make known thy faithfulness to all generations."*

Romans 8:28 *"And we know that all things work together for Good to them that love God, to them who are the called according to his purpose."*

Jeremiah 29:11 *"For I know the thoughts that I think toward you, saith the Lord, thoughts of peace, and not of evil, to give you an expected end."*

Mark 10:27 *"And Jesus looking upon them saith, with men it is impossible, but not with God: for with God all things are possible."*

Healing Habits for a Healthy You

Part Four

Healing Habits for a Healthy You

Rest. *Sleep requirements are based on your age; however, the older you are the less sleep is required. Adults require at least 6 hours of sleep per twenty-four hour period, up to a maximum of 8 hours of sleep. Lack of sleep can affect a person's metabolism, livelihood, mind process and immune system.*

Eat Well. *Adults need 6 small meals per day, or 3 good variation meals per day. Everyone must eat to survive; however, it's what we eat that makes us what and who we are.*

Brush Your Teeth. *Teeth brushing and flossing is essential. Brush your teeth after you eat. Brushing and Flossing will often prevent you from becoming sick. Not everything we place in our mouths is clean or free of germs. Our mouths allow germs into our bodies that toothpaste and floss can destory.*

Stay Active. *It's true; people who work until they are old and gray live longer. Activity keeps people healthy while activating metabolism and the immune system. Find something you enjoy and stick to it.*

Prayer and Meditation. Alone Time. *Every day we need time to reflect, think and pray about life's obstacles. Ever have a day that you don't have a second to yourself and you feel overwhelmed? If you are a busy mom or dad, bathroom time is a great way to get alone with no one bothering you. Try to make time for yourself every day to just breathe, think, pray and deal with the day's events. Throw a fit if you need to. Plan what time will work best and set aside time in your schedule to be alone. Learning to self-reflect and have alone time is healthy. Sometimes it is just a matter of finding the time to do so.*

Love. Love to be loved. *We must live to love in order to feel as if we are a part of this life. Think of how newborns need to bond with their mothers in order to have a healthy attachment style. Newborns who lack motherly bonding upon birth show signs of insecurity from the lack of bonding. Smile and know you are like everyone else—a human being. We all make mistakes, live and learn, and must love to be loved.*

Laugh. *Did you know that laughing is good for you? Laughing burns calories. If you haven't laughed in a while, go to YouTube and search for funny videos. Find what makes you laugh. Maybe no one else understands your humor, but that is okay. If it makes you laugh, that's a good thing.*

Positive Surroundings. *If you can find who and what makes you feel positive—cling to it. Do not cling to other people because that can possibly push them away and cause a source of positive energy to change to negative. Choose your surroundings carefully. Learn to feel your emotions and identify them. When you know what you feel and can name it, you can stay clear of negativity and keep yourself positive.*

Just Live. *Sometimes we need to just live and not put standards, boundaries or expectations on ourselves. Rules can cause stress in our own lives and the lives of others around us. Remember, we want to be healthy while assisting others to be healthy and sometimes that means relax and live life. If we ourselves can become healthy, then we can reach out and help others in become healthy.*

Heather Briley Bynog, BSN, RN

Also by Angelena Cortello

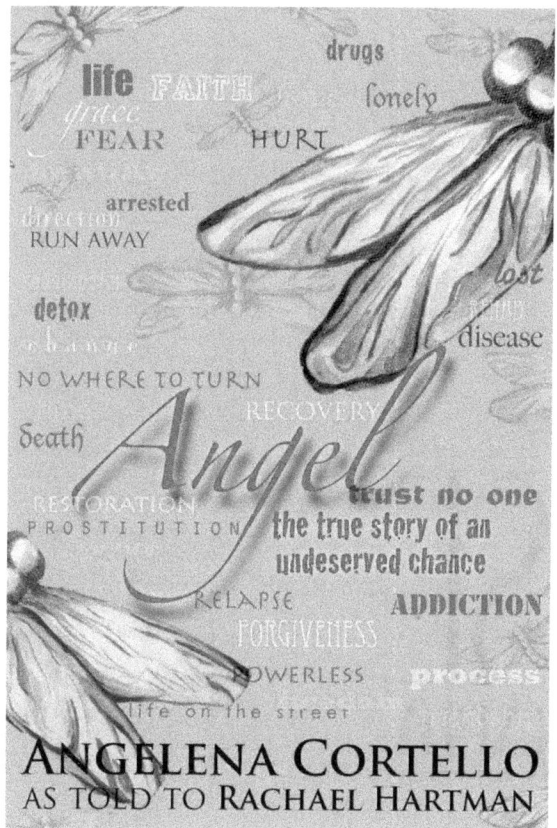

Angel: The True Story of an Undeserved Chance

Angel Cortello was lost in a world of emotional problems, addiction, prostitution and the street life. This is the true story of how she chose recovery and freedom, even in the midst of consequences such as HIV.

"You don't have to live your life like this," he said. He put a wad of cash on the bed, handed me the key to the hotel room and walked out. I never saw the man again.

…He could see something in me that I couldn't see in myself. He could see someone better than who I had become…

A dramatic narrative that reads like a novel, Angel Cortello shares her testimony of healing and hope and life lessons she's learned since finding freedom and beginning recovery.

Available through all major book retailers:
Barnes & Noble, Amazon, Kindle

Or directly from
angelcortello.com or **ourwrittenlives.com**

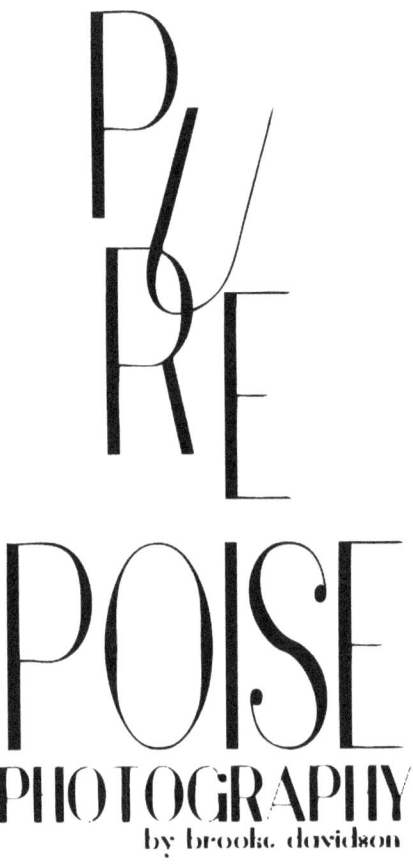

Check out
"Pure Poise Photography by Brooke Davidson"
on Facebook!

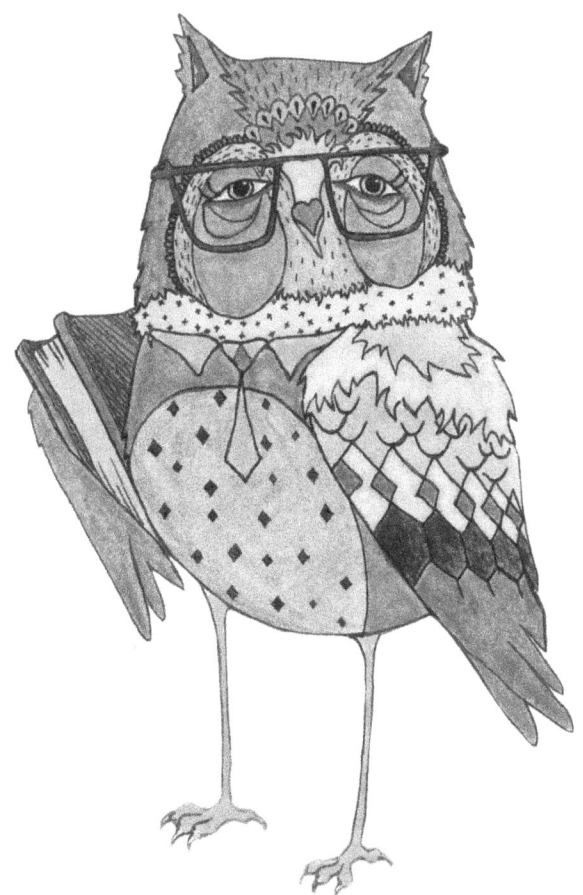

Our Written Lives
book publishing services
www.owlofhope.com

www.ingramcontent.com/pod-product-compliance
Lightning Source LLC
Chambersburg PA
CBHW081157020426
42333CB00020B/2534